THE HERBAL MEDICINE & NATURAL REMEDIES BIBLE

[15 in 1] The Complete Guide of Healing Herbs for ALL Diseases.

Crafting Herbal Remedies, Essential Oils, Infusions, Tea, etc. in Easy Way.

Copyright 2023 by Drina Kaulja

TABLE OF CONTENT

1. Foundations of Herbal Medicine: An Introduction to Healing Plants

Chapter 1: History of Herbal Medicine: A Journey Through Time

Throughout the annals of human history, the use of herbs and plants as remedies for various ailments has been a constant thread, weaving its way through cultures and civilizations across the globe. This chapter embarks on a journey through time to explore the rich history of herbal medicine, tracing its origins, evolution, and enduring significance in human healthcare.

Ancient Beginnings

The roots of herbal medicine can be traced back to the earliest human societies. In prehistoric times, our ancestors relied on their innate knowledge of the natural world to identify plants with medicinal properties. The first documented evidence of herbal medicine dates back over 5,000 years to the Sumerians, who recorded their use of herbs on clay tablets.

Ancient Egypt and China

One of the most well-known ancient civilizations that extensively practiced herbal medicine was ancient Egypt. The Ebers Papyrus, a medical text from around 1500 BCE, contains detailed information on various medicinal plants, showcasing the Egyptians' advanced understanding of herbs and their healing properties. Similarly, ancient Chinese medicine, rooted in the teachings of the Yellow Emperor's Inner Canon (Huangdi Neijing), has a rich tradition of using herbs to restore balance and promote health.

Greece and Rome

In classical antiquity, the Greeks and Romans made significant contributions to the development of herbal medicine. The Greek physician Hippocrates, often regarded as the father of Western medicine, emphasized the importance of using natural remedies, including herbs, to treat diseases. His works laid the foundation for the use of herbs in the Hippocratic tradition. The Roman naturalist Pliny the Elder documented hundreds of medicinal plants in his "Naturalis Historia," further advancing the understanding of herbal remedies in the ancient world.

Middle Ages and Herbalism

During the Middle Ages, herbalism thrived in Europe, with monasteries serving as centers of knowledge and preservation of herbal lore. Monastic herbalists cultivated and studied medicinal plants, compiling manuscripts known as "herbals" that provided detailed descriptions and instructions for their use. The works of notable herbalists like Hildegard of Bingen and Nicholas Culpeper are still referenced today.

The Renaissance and Beyond

The Renaissance marked a period of renewed interest in classical knowledge, including herbal medicine. Herbals, such as John Gerard's "The Herball" and Nicholas Culpeper's "The English Physician," became influential texts during this time. The discovery of the New World expanded the repertoire of medicinal plants available to European herbalists.

Modernization and Challenges

With the advent of modern medicine in the 19th and 20th centuries, herbalism faced challenges as it clashed with the emerging pharmaceutical industry. However, herbal medicine never disappeared entirely. In recent decades, there has been a resurgence of interest in herbal remedies, driven by a desire for natural and holistic approaches to healthcare.

The Global Impact of Herbal Medicine

Herbal medicine has left an indelible mark on cultures worldwide, each contributing its unique insights and practices. In India, Ayurveda, an ancient healing system, incorporates a vast array of herbs and botanicals to balance the body's doshas. Native American traditions have long relied on indigenous plants for healing, with a profound understanding of the natural world's interconnectedness. Similarly, African traditional medicine encompasses a wide range of herbal remedies passed down through generations.

Scientific Advancements and Validation

In recent times, herbal medicine has gained renewed credibility through scientific research and validation. Modern laboratories have identified active compounds within plants, explaining their medicinal properties. For example, the discovery of artemisinin from Artemisia annua, a plant used in traditional Chinese medicine, revolutionized the treatment of malaria. Herbal medicine is increasingly integrated into mainstream healthcare, and its potential benefits are being explored for a wide range of conditions, from chronic diseases to mental health.

Cultural and Ethical Considerations

The practice of herbal medicine is not merely a matter of identifying active compounds but also deeply intertwined with cultural and ethical considerations. Indigenous knowledge and traditional healing practices must be respected and protected, especially in the face of biopiracy and exploitation of medicinal plants. The equitable sharing of benefits from herbal resources is an ongoing global challenge.

Herbal Medicine Today

In contemporary times, herbal medicine thrives as a complementary and alternative form of healthcare. Many individuals seek herbal remedies for various reasons, including a desire for holistic approaches, concerns about side effects associated with pharmaceutical drugs, and a growing preference for sustainable and eco-friendly healthcare options. Herbalists, naturopathic physicians, and integrative medicine practitioners are working alongside conventional healthcare providers, offering a diverse range of treatments that often combine modern medical knowledge with traditional herbal wisdom.

Challenges and Future Prospects

Despite its resurgence, herbal medicine faces challenges related to standardization, quality control, and regulation. Ensuring the safety and efficacy of herbal products is a priority. Additionally, as herbal medicine continues to evolve, ongoing research is needed to validate its claims and optimize treatment protocols. Integrating herbal medicine into the broader healthcare system while respecting cultural diversity and ecological sustainability remains a complex endeavor.

The Science of Herbal Medicine

The study of herbal medicine has evolved significantly over time, blending traditional knowledge with rigorous scientific investigation. Phytochemistry, the branch of science that focuses on the chemical composition of plants, has played a crucial role in uncovering the active compounds responsible for the therapeutic effects of herbs. Researchers employ advanced techniques such as chromatography and mass spectrometry to isolate and identify these bioactive compounds. This scientific approach has led to the development of standardized herbal extracts and a deeper understanding of how herbs interact with the body at the molecular level.

Holistic Healing and Herbalism

Herbal medicine operates on the principle of holistic healing, emphasizing the interconnectedness of mind, body, and spirit. This approach goes beyond symptom management, aiming to address the root causes of illness. Herbalists often consider individual constitution, emotional well-being, and lifestyle factors when creating treatment plans. The holistic perspective recognizes that health is not just the absence of disease but a state of balance and vitality.

Herbal Medicine in Practice

Practitioners of herbal medicine draw from an extensive repertoire of herbs, each with its unique properties and applications. Herbs can be administered in various forms, including teas, tinctures, capsules, and topical preparations. Combining herbs into formulas is a common practice to synergistically enhance their therapeutic effects. Herbalists tailor treatments to individual needs, taking into account factors such as the patient's specific condition, age, and overall health.

Herbs and Modern Healthcare

In recent years, herbal medicine has gained acceptance within conventional healthcare systems. Many pharmaceutical drugs have their origins in plants, underscoring the value of traditional herbal knowledge. Some herbs, like St. John's Wort and Echinacea, are well-studied for their efficacy in managing conditions such as depression and immune support, respectively. Integrative medicine centers and hospitals increasingly offer herbal therapies as part of comprehensive patient care.

Research and Evidence-Based Practice

The field of herbal medicine continues to evolve through rigorous scientific research. Clinical trials, systematic reviews, and meta-analyses are conducted to evaluate the safety and effectiveness of herbal treatments. Organizations like the World Health Organization (WHO) and the National Institutes of Health (NIH) provide guidelines and funding for herbal research. Evidence-based practice in herbal medicine helps bridge the gap between traditional wisdom and modern healthcare standards.

Cultural Diversity and Sustainability

Cultural diversity plays a significant role in herbal medicine, with each culture bringing its unique knowledge and practices to the field. Indigenous communities worldwide maintain a wealth of herbal wisdom passed down through generations. Preserving and respecting these diverse traditions while ensuring the sustainable harvesting of medicinal plants is a critical aspect of herbalism's future.

The Continuing Journey of Herbal Medicine

The journey of herbal medicine through history, science, and practice is an ongoing exploration. As humanity faces new health challenges and seeks more sustainable and holistic approaches to well-being, herbal medicine remains a dynamic and relevant field. Its capacity to adapt, integrate scientific advancements, and honor cultural traditions makes herbal medicine a valuable asset in the ever-evolving landscape of healthcare. In the chapters ahead, we will delve deeper into specific herbs, their therapeutic applications, and the best practices for incorporating herbal remedies into a modern wellness routine.

Chapter 2: Why Choose Herbal Medicine? Benefits and Limitations

The Benefits of Herbal Medicine

Natural Healing: One of the primary reasons people choose herbal medicine is its natural approach to healing. Herbal remedies are derived from plants, making them generally gentler on the body and associated with fewer side effects compared to synthetic pharmaceuticals.

Holistic Approach: Herbal medicine embraces a holistic perspective on health, addressing not only physical symptoms but also considering emotional and mental well-being. It aims to restore balance and harmony in the body, promoting overall wellness.

Individualized Treatment: Herbalists often tailor treatments to individual needs, taking into account factors such as the patient's constitution, lifestyle, and specific health condition. This personalized approach can lead to more effective and well-tolerated therapies.

Ancient Wisdom: Herbal medicine has a rich history dating back thousands of years. It draws on the accumulated knowledge and wisdom of diverse cultures, offering a time-tested approach to healing that has withstood the test of time.

Wide Range of Applications: Herbs offer a vast array of therapeutic possibilities. They can be used to address a wide range of health concerns, from common colds and digestive issues to chronic conditions like arthritis and anxiety.

Complementary to Modern Medicine: Herbal medicine can complement conventional medical treatments. Many pharmaceutical drugs have their origins in plant compounds, and herbal remedies can be used alongside prescription medications, sometimes reducing the need for higher doses of synthetic drugs.

Limitations of Herbal Medicine

Limited Scientific Evidence: While there is a growing body of scientific research supporting the efficacy of certain herbs, not all herbal remedies have been extensively studied. This lack of scientific evidence can lead to uncertainty about their effectiveness.

Varied Quality and Potency: Herbal products on the market can vary widely in quality and potency. Inconsistent sourcing, processing, and labeling can make it challenging to ensure that you are getting a high-quality product.

Interaction with Medications: Some herbs can interact with prescription medications, potentially causing adverse effects or diminishing the drugs' effectiveness. It is crucial to consult with a healthcare professional when combining herbal remedies with pharmaceuticals.

Safety Concerns: While herbs are generally considered safe, they are not entirely without risk. Allergic reactions, side effects, and toxicities can occur, particularly if herbs are used improperly or in excessive amounts.

Slow Acting: Herbal remedies often work gradually, addressing the root causes of health issues rather than providing quick relief. This slower onset of action may not be suitable for acute conditions that require immediate intervention.

Cultural and Ethical Considerations: The sourcing of certain herbs may raise ethical and sustainability concerns. Overharvesting and habitat destruction can threaten some plant species, emphasizing the need for responsible and sustainable practices.

Additional Considerations for Choosing Herbal Medicine

Preventative Health: Herbal medicine is not solely about treating illness; it also plays a role in preventing health issues. Many herbs possess immune-boosting, antioxidant, and anti-inflammatory properties, making them valuable for maintaining overall well-being and reducing the risk of chronic diseases.

Empowerment and Self-Care: Herbal medicine empowers individuals to take an active role in their health and well-being. Learning about herbs and their uses can promote a sense of self-sufficiency and self-care, allowing people to make informed choices about their health.

Minimal Environmental Impact: In comparison to the pharmaceutical industry, herbal medicine production often has a lower environmental footprint. Cultivating and harvesting medicinal plants can be done sustainably, reducing the carbon footprint associated with drug manufacturing.

Cultural Connection: For some, choosing herbal medicine is a way to connect with their cultural heritage. Many cultures have deep roots in herbalism, and embracing these traditions can foster a sense of cultural identity and pride.

Navigating the Complexities of Herbal Medicine

Educational Resources: To make informed choices in herbal medicine, it's essential to access reliable educational resources. Books, courses, and consultations with trained herbalists can provide valuable knowledge and guidance.

Collaborative Healthcare: Integrating herbal medicine into your healthcare routine can be done in collaboration with conventional healthcare providers. Open communication with your doctors ensures that all treatments, whether herbal or pharmaceutical, work together safely and effectively.

Trial and Observation: Herbal medicine often involves a degree of trial and observation. Each person's response to herbs can vary, and it may take some time to find the most suitable remedies and dosages.

Regulatory Oversight: Be aware of the regulatory framework governing herbal products in your region. Some countries have robust regulations, while others may have limited oversight. Choose products from reputable manufacturers and suppliers to ensure quality and safety.

The Future of Herbal Medicine

As herbal medicine continues to evolve, there is a growing interest in scientific validation, standardization, and evidence-based practice. Research into the safety and efficacy of herbs is ongoing, offering the potential for more widespread acceptance and integration into mainstream healthcare.

Emerging Trends in Herbal Medicine

Modern Research and Validation: The integration of herbal medicine into the modern healthcare system is increasingly supported by rigorous scientific research. Clinical trials, molecular studies, and pharmacological investigations are shedding light on the mechanisms of action of various herbs, offering evidence-based validation for their use.

Herbal Formulations: Modern herbalists and manufacturers are developing innovative herbal formulations that combine multiple herbs to enhance therapeutic effects. These formulations are often designed to address complex health issues and promote synergy among the herbs used.

Herbal Supplements: The availability of herbal supplements in various forms, including capsules, tinctures, and powders, has made herbal medicine more accessible and convenient. These products are standardized to contain specific concentrations of active compounds, ensuring consistent dosing.

Herbs in Functional Medicine: Functional medicine practitioners are increasingly incorporating herbal remedies into their holistic approach. Herbs are seen as tools for addressing underlying imbalances and optimizing bodily functions, aligning with the principles of functional medicine.

Herbal Medicine for Mental Health: The role of herbs in mental health is gaining recognition. Many herbs, such as St. John's Wort and ashwagandha, have demonstrated potential benefits in managing conditions like depression, anxiety, and stress. This area of herbal medicine is undergoing significant exploration.

Community and Global Impact

Community Herbalism: Community-based herbalism is on the rise, with local herbalists and herbal gardens offering educational resources and herbal remedies. This grassroots movement fosters a sense of community, self-reliance, and resilience in health.

Global Exchange of Herbal Knowledge: The globalization of herbal knowledge allows for the exchange of traditions and practices from different cultures. This cross-cultural sharing enriches the field of herbal medicine and broadens its therapeutic possibilities.

Sustainable Practices: Recognizing the importance of preserving herbal resources, sustainable harvesting practices are gaining prominence. Wildcrafting guidelines and ethical cultivation methods are being developed to protect both plant species and ecosystems.

Personal Empowerment and Well-Being

Personalized Wellness Plans: With herbal medicine, individuals can take an active role in crafting personalized wellness plans. By understanding their unique health needs and incorporating herbs accordingly, people can proactively manage their health.

Preventive Healthcare: Herbal medicine's emphasis on prevention aligns with the growing interest in preventive healthcare. Many herbs are used proactively to boost immunity, support digestion, and maintain overall well-being.

Complementary and Integrative Healthcare: Herbal medicine's acceptance as a complementary or integrative healthcare approach is likely to continue to grow. Collaboration between herbalists and conventional healthcare providers can lead to more comprehensive and patient-centered care.

Chapter 3: Key Principles of Herbal Medicine

Holism and Balance

At the core of herbal medicine lies the principle of holism, which recognizes that the body is an interconnected system of physical, emotional, and mental aspects. Herbalists view health as a state of balance and harmony within this holistic framework. When illness occurs, it is often seen as a manifestation of imbalances in the body, and herbal remedies are employed to restore equilibrium.

Herbalists consider not only the physical symptoms but also the emotional and mental well-being of an individual. The goal is not merely to alleviate symptoms but to address the root causes of the ailment and promote overall wellness.

Individualization of Treatment

No two individuals are exactly alike, and herbal medicine acknowledges this uniqueness. Herbalists emphasize the importance of individualized treatment plans. Factors such as a person's constitution, genetics, lifestyle, and specific health condition are carefully considered when selecting and prescribing herbs.

This personalized approach ensures that the chosen herbal remedies are most suitable for the individual's needs and are likely to be well-tolerated. It recognizes that what works for one person may not work the same way for another.

Healing from Nature

Herbal medicine is grounded in the idea that nature provides an abundance of healing resources. Plants, with their complex chemical compositions, offer a diverse array of therapeutic compounds. Herbalists harness the power of nature's pharmacy by identifying, selecting, and preparing herbs to address various health concerns.

The use of whole plants or specific plant parts (leaves, roots, flowers, etc.) and the choice of preparation methods (teas, tinctures, poultices) are guided by the knowledge of how each plant interacts with the body.

Prevention and Maintenance of Health

Herbal medicine places a strong emphasis on preventive healthcare. Herbs are not just utilized for the treatment of acute illnesses; they are also used proactively to maintain and promote good health. Many herbs possess immune-boosting, antioxidant, and adaptogenic properties that support the body's natural defense mechanisms.

This preventive approach aligns with the idea of wellness as an ongoing process, rather than simply the absence of disease. By incorporating herbs into daily routines, individuals can bolster their overall well-being.

Respect for Cultural Traditions

The practice of herbal medicine is deeply rooted in cultural traditions worldwide. Different cultures have developed their unique systems of herbal knowledge and healing practices. Herbalists respect and honor these traditions, recognizing the valuable contributions they make to the field.

The global exchange of herbal knowledge allows for cross-cultural learning and enrichment. It fosters an appreciation of the diverse uses of herbs and their cultural significance.

Safety and Ethical Considerations

Safety is a paramount concern in herbal medicine. While herbs are generally considered safe when used appropriately, it is crucial to be aware of potential interactions with medications, allergies, and contraindications. Herbalists are trained to assess individual health histories and make informed choices regarding herbal treatments.

Ethical considerations also come into play, particularly with regards to sustainable harvesting and sourcing of herbs. Responsible practices, such as wildcrafting guidelines and ethical cultivation, help ensure the long-term availability of medicinal plants.

Ongoing Learning and Research

The field of herbal medicine is dynamic and continuously evolving. Herbalists engage in ongoing learning and research to stay informed about the latest developments. This includes keeping abreast of scientific studies, new herbal discoveries, and emerging applications of traditional herbs.

By staying updated, herbalists can offer the most effective and evidence-based treatments to their clients, incorporating the latest research into their practice.

Observation and Assessment

A fundamental skill in herbal medicine is the ability to keenly observe and assess the patient. Herbalists often start by taking a detailed medical history and conducting a thorough physical examination. This process involves not only identifying symptoms but also understanding their underlying causes and patterns.

Observation extends beyond the physical realm. Herbalists pay attention to a patient's emotional state, energy levels, and overall constitution. These subtle cues aid in the selection of herbs that resonate with the individual's specific needs.

The Vital Role of Plant Constituents

Each herb contains a complex mix of chemical constituents that contribute to its therapeutic properties. Herbalists delve into the intricate chemistry of plants to understand how these constituents interact with the body. This knowledge guides the selection of herbs and determines the most suitable form of preparation.

Different plant parts, such as leaves, roots, and flowers, may contain distinct concentrations of active compounds. Additionally, the choice of preparation methods, such as decoctions, infusions, or tinctures, can influence the bioavailability and effectiveness of these constituents.

Synergy and Formulations

Herbal medicine often relies on the concept of synergy, where combining multiple herbs enhances their therapeutic effects. Herbalists carefully craft formulations, selecting herbs that complement and potentiate each other's actions. This synergistic approach is akin to orchestrating a symphony of healing within the body.

Formulations may target specific health conditions or systems in the body, offering a holistic approach to treatment. The art of formulation is a hallmark of herbal medicine, and herbalists use their knowledge to create balanced and effective remedies.

Responsiveness and Adaptability

Herbal medicine embraces the idea that each person's health needs can change over time. Herbalists remain responsive to their patients' evolving conditions and adapt treatments accordingly. This adaptability allows for ongoing refinement of herbal protocols to align with the patient's progress.

Moreover, the dynamic nature of herbs means that their effects can vary among individuals. Herbalists are prepared to modify treatment plans as needed, fine-tuning dosage, herb selection, and formulation to optimize results.

Integration with Conventional Medicine

While herbal medicine is a distinct practice, it can coexist harmoniously with conventional medicine. Collaboration between herbalists and healthcare providers is increasingly common, as both recognize the value of integrating different modalities for patient care.

Herbalists work to ensure that herbal treatments do not interfere with medications or treatments prescribed by medical doctors. This collaborative approach acknowledges the strengths of both systems and prioritizes the patient's well-being.

Empowerment and Education

A fundamental principle of herbal medicine is to empower individuals to take an active role in their health. Herbalists educate their patients about the herbs they are using, providing information on dosages, potential side effects, and expected outcomes.

This educational aspect extends to promoting self-care practices. Patients are encouraged to make lifestyle changes, dietary adjustments, and herbal supplementation choices that support their health goals. By fostering self-awareness and knowledge, herbal medicine empowers individuals to be active participants in their healing journey.

Traditional Wisdom and Lineage

Herbal medicine often draws from generations of traditional wisdom and lineage. Many herbalists inherit knowledge and practices from their mentors, family members, or cultural backgrounds. This lineage carries not only the accumulated herbal knowledge but also the values, ethics, and cultural significance of herbal traditions.

Traditional wisdom informs the selection of herbs, preparation methods, and the understanding of local ecosystems. It respects the wisdom passed down through generations and maintains a connection to ancestral healing practices.

Herbal Energetics and Constitutions

Herbalists consider the energetics of herbs and their compatibility with an individual's constitution.

Energetics refer to the inherent qualities of herbs, such as hot, cold, damp, or dry. These qualities are used to match herbs to a person's constitution, which is their unique combination of physical and emotional traits.

For example, a person with a "cold" constitution may benefit from warming herbs to balance their system, while someone with a "hot" constitution might find relief from cooling herbs. Understanding these dynamics enhances the precision of herbal prescribing.

Seasonal and Environmental Awareness

Herbal medicine is attuned to the seasons and the environment. Different herbs thrive at specific times of the year, and their therapeutic properties can vary with seasonal changes. Herbalists take advantage of these variations, using herbs that align with the seasons to support overall health.

Furthermore, environmental awareness is integral to herbalism. Sustainable harvesting practices, ethical wildcrafting, and organic cultivation methods are employed to protect herbal resources and preserve natural ecosystems.

Personal Connection with Plants

Many herbalists develop a deep personal connection with the plants they work with. This connection often involves spending time in nature, observing plant growth, and fostering a sense of reverence for the plant world. Herbalists may even engage in practices like plant meditation or spirit journeys to enhance their understanding of plants' healing qualities.

This personal connection with plants goes beyond their chemical constituents; it is a spiritual and intuitive relationship that enriches the herbalist's practice.

The Continual Learning Journey

Herbal medicine is a lifelong learning journey. Herbalists recognize that there is always more to discover, and they remain open to new knowledge and experiences. Whether through attending workshops, conducting their research, or exchanging insights with other herbalists, the pursuit of knowledge is ongoing.

This commitment to continual learning ensures that herbalists stay current with emerging herbal discoveries and evolving healthcare practices.

Chapter 4: Deciphering Plant Parts and Their Uses

In the world of herbal medicine, understanding the various plant parts and their specific uses is a fundamental aspect. Each part of a plant, be it the roots, leaves, flowers, seeds, or bark, possesses unique properties and therapeutic potential. In this chapter, we will explore these plant parts and how they are utilized in herbal remedies.

Roots

Roots are a vital plant part used extensively in herbal medicine. They are known for their grounding and anchoring qualities. Roots often contain concentrated compounds, making them valuable for their therapeutic effects.

Examples: Ginseng, Echinacea, Valerian, Licorice

Uses: Roots are used for a range of purposes, including immune support, stress reduction, and digestive health. They are commonly employed to address conditions related to the lower body, such as the digestive system and the musculoskeletal system.

Leaves

Leaves are among the most commonly used plant parts in herbal remedies. They are often rich in essential oils, chlorophyll, and other bioactive compounds.

Examples: Peppermint, Sage, Eucalyptus, Nettles

Uses: Leaves have diverse applications, such as promoting digestion, soothing respiratory issues, and supporting the nervous system. They are also used for their antimicrobial and anti-inflammatory properties.

Flowers

Flowers are prized for their beauty and fragrant aromas, but they also have therapeutic value. They are often associated with uplifting and soothing qualities.

Examples: Chamomile, Lavender, Rose

Uses: Flowers are commonly used to relieve stress, anxiety, and sleep disturbances. They can be prepared as teas, infused oils, or incorporated into bath products for their calming effects.

Seeds

Seeds are packed with nutrients and essential oils. They are often used for their potential to support digestion, provide essential fatty acids, and deliver concentrated nutrients.

Examples: Flaxseeds, Fenugreek, Chia seeds

Uses: Seeds can be used to promote digestive health, address hormonal imbalances, and provide a source of dietary fiber and healthy fats. They are also used for their potential to support cardiovascular health.

Bark

Bark is a less commonly used plant part in herbal medicine, but it can be highly valuable due to its concentration of bioactive compounds. Bark is typically harvested from mature trees.

Examples: White Willow Bark, Cinnamon, Slippery Elm

Uses: Bark is often used for its anti-inflammatory and analgesic properties. It can be employed in remedies for conditions like pain, digestive discomfort, and respiratory issues.

Berries and Fruits

Berries and fruits are cherished for their delicious flavors and vibrant colors. They are rich in vitamins, antioxidants, and other beneficial compounds.

Examples: Elderberries, Hawthorn Berries, Cranberries

Uses: Berries and fruits are often used to support the immune system, promote heart health, and address urinary tract issues. They are also incorporated into culinary recipes and beverages for their taste and nutritional value.

Stems and Shoots

Stems and young shoots are less commonly used in herbal medicine but still offer therapeutic potential. They are often harvested when tender and may be used in specific remedies.

Examples: Asparagus shoots, Horsetail

Uses: Stems and shoots are sometimes employed for their diuretic properties and as a source of minerals. Horsetail, for example, is used to support bone health due to its silica content.

Whole Plant

In some cases, the entire plant, including various parts such as leaves, stems, and flowers, is used in herbal medicine. This approach harnesses the synergistic effects of all plant components.

Examples: Plantain, Yarrow, Dandelion

Uses: Whole plants can have a broad range of applications, including wound healing, detoxification, and digestive support. They are often used for their versatility and comprehensive therapeutic potential.

Rhizomes and Tubers

Rhizomes and tubers are underground stems or root-like structures that store energy and nutrients for the plant. They often have a starchy or fibrous texture and are used for their nourishing and grounding qualities.

Examples: Turmeric, Ginger, Burdock

Uses: Rhizomes and tubers are known for their anti-inflammatory properties and digestive benefits. They are commonly used to soothe digestive discomfort, reduce inflammation, and support overall wellness.

Aerial Parts

The aerial parts of a plant include everything above the ground, such as leaves, flowers, and stems. When harvested together, they provide a holistic representation of the plant's therapeutic potential.

Examples: St. John's Wort, Lemon Balm, Oregano

Uses: Aerial parts are versatile and can be used for a range of purposes, including mood support, relaxation, and immune system enhancement. They are often employed in teas, tinctures, and topical preparations.

Resin and Gums

Resins and gums are sticky substances exuded by certain trees and plants. They contain volatile compounds and are used for their antimicrobial and soothing properties.

Examples: Frankincense, Myrrh, Copal

Uses: Resins and gums are traditionally used in incense and as topical preparations for wound healing and skin care. They are also valued for their potential to support respiratory health.

Lichen

Lichens are unique organisms resulting from a symbiotic relationship between fungi and algae or cyanobacteria. They are used less frequently in herbal medicine but have historical and cultural significance.

Examples: Usnea, Iceland Moss

Uses: Lichens are often used for their antimicrobial properties and are employed in remedies for respiratory issues and immune support. Usnea, for example, is known as "old man's beard" and is used to address throat and lung concerns.

Sap and Latex

Sap and latex are fluids that flow within a plant's vascular system. While not commonly used in herbal medicine, they have been employed historically for their therapeutic properties.

Examples: Aloe Vera (latex), Gum Arabic (sap)

Uses: Aloe Vera latex is sometimes used for its laxative effects, while gum arabic (acacia gum) is employed in various industries, including food, pharmaceuticals, and cosmetics.

Non-Plant Materials

In some traditional herbal practices, non-plant materials like minerals and metals are also included. These materials are used sparingly and often in specialized preparations.

Examples: Gold, Silver, Sulfur

Uses: Non-plant materials are usually used in highly diluted forms known as homeopathic remedies. They are believed to have subtle yet profound effects on the body's energetic and physical balance.

Understanding the diverse range of plant parts and other materials used in herbal medicine allows herbalists to create tailored remedies for a wide array of health concerns. By selecting the most appropriate plant parts and preparations, herbalists can harness the full potential of nature's healing resources. In the chapters ahead, we will explore specific herbs in greater detail, examining their plant parts and preparation methods to gain a deeper understanding of how they can be used effectively in herbal medicine.

Fungi and Mycelium

While not plants, fungi play a significant role in herbal medicine, particularly in traditional Chinese medicine and mycology. The fruiting bodies (mushrooms) and mycelium (the underground network) of fungi contain various bioactive compounds with therapeutic potential.

Examples: Reishi Mushroom, Cordyceps, Turkey Tail

Uses: Fungi are known for their immune-modulating effects, adaptogenic properties, and potential to support vitality. They are often used to boost the immune system, enhance endurance, and address various health concerns.

Bulbs

Bulbs are underground storage organs that store energy and nutrients for the plant. They are often used in herbal medicine for their grounding and nourishing qualities.

Examples: Garlic, Onion, Daffodil (used in homeopathy)

Uses: Bulbs like garlic are renowned for their antimicrobial properties and cardiovascular support. They are also used in culinary dishes and sometimes as remedies for respiratory and digestive health.

Whole Plant Combinations

In some cases, herbalists use combinations of various plant parts from the same plant. This approach capitalizes on the synergistic effects of different plant components.

Examples: Holy Basil (Tulsi), Milk Thistle, Comfrey

Uses: Whole plant combinations provide comprehensive support for specific health concerns. Holy Basil, for instance, combines leaves, stems, and flowers and is used for stress relief, immune support, and general well-being.

Metabolites and Extracts

In modern herbal medicine, scientists extract specific metabolites or compounds from plants for therapeutic purposes. These extracts are often standardized to contain specific active constituents.

Examples: Echinacea extract, Ginkgo biloba extract, Curcumin (from Turmeric)

Uses: Extracts offer concentrated and consistent doses of bioactive compounds, making them suitable for research-backed herbal treatments. They are used for various health issues, including immune support, cognitive health, and inflammation.

Animal-Derived Substances

While less common, animal-derived substances are occasionally used in traditional and folk herbal medicine. These substances may be employed in specialized formulations.

Examples: Royal Jelly (bee product), Pearl powder (from crushed pearls)

Uses: Animal-derived substances are believed to provide unique nutritional and therapeutic benefits. Royal Jelly is used for its potential to support overall vitality and well-being, while pearl powder is used in traditional Chinese medicine for skin health and longevity.

Understanding the wide range of plant parts, fungi, extracts, and even animal-derived substances used in herbal medicine highlights the diversity of therapeutic possibilities within this field. Herbalists carefully select and combine these elements to create remedies tailored to individual health needs. In the following chapters, we will explore specific herbs and their applications, considering the diverse array of plant parts and preparations that contribute to their healing potential.

Chapter 5: Cultivating a Herbal Mindset: Ethics and Sustainability

In the practice of herbal medicine, ethics and sustainability are integral components of a responsible and holistic approach. Cultivating a herbal mindset that prioritizes ethical considerations and sustainable practices ensures the well-being of both individuals and the planet. This chapter delves into the principles and practices that guide ethical herbalism and sustainable use of medicinal plants.

Respect for Plant Communities

Ethical herbalism begins with a deep respect for plant communities. Herbalists understand that plants are not merely resources but living beings that play critical roles in ecosystems. This respect extends to wild plants and cultivated herbs alike.

Wildcrafting: When harvesting wild plants, herbalists adhere to ethical wildcrafting practices. They minimize their impact on plant populations, avoid overharvesting, and follow guidelines for sustainable harvesting set by organizations and experts.

Cultivation: In cultivated herb gardens, herbalists strive for sustainable and organic practices. They consider factors like soil health, companion planting, and biodiversity to support thriving plant communities.

Sustainable Harvesting Practices

Sustainability is a core principle in herbal medicine. Herbalists recognize that responsible harvesting ensures the long-term availability of medicinal plants.

Harvesting Ethics: Herbalists follow ethical guidelines when harvesting plants. They avoid taking more than what is needed, leave no trace in the wild, and ensure minimal disruption to ecosystems.

Regenerative Agriculture: In cultivated settings, herbalists may engage in regenerative agriculture practices, which aim to restore and enhance the health of the land and soil while growing medicinal herbs.

Conservation Efforts

Many herbalists actively participate in conservation efforts to protect endangered plant species and their habitats.

At-Risk Plants: Ethical herbalists are aware of plants listed as at-risk or endangered and avoid using them in their remedies. They support initiatives that aim to conserve these species.

Cultivation of Threatened Plants: Herbalists may grow threatened plants in gardens or collaborate with conservation organizations to cultivate and propagate them, contributing to their preservation.

Responsible Sourcing

When purchasing herbs and herbal products, ethical herbalists prioritize responsible sourcing. They support companies that adhere to sustainable and ethical practices.

Fair Trade: Ethical herbalists may choose products certified as fair trade, ensuring that workers involved in herb cultivation and processing receive fair wages and working conditions.

Quality and Transparency: They prioritize products with transparent labeling, clear information on sourcing, and adherence to quality control standards.

Avoidance of Over-Harvested Species

Herbalists are conscientious about the plants they use in their remedies. They avoid over-harvested species, helping prevent further depletion of these valuable resources.

Substitutes: When a popular herb is over-harvested, herbalists seek suitable substitutes or alternatives to reduce pressure on the at-risk plant.

Sustainable Preparation Methods

Ethical herbalists choose preparation methods that minimize waste and environmental impact.

Low-Impact Processing: They may prefer methods like tinctures and infusions, which use minimal energy and produce less waste compared to other extraction methods.

Cultural Respect

Ethical herbalism respects the cultural significance of plant medicine. Herbalists acknowledge and honor the traditional knowledge and practices of Indigenous communities and other cultures.

Cultural Appropriation: They avoid cultural appropriation by seeking permission and guidance from Indigenous elders or knowledge keepers when working with plants from specific cultural traditions.

Education and Advocacy

Ethical herbalists are advocates for sustainable practices and ethical considerations in the field of herbal medicine.

Public Awareness: They educate the public about responsible herbal practices, conservation efforts, and the importance of ethical sourcing.

Policy Advocacy: Some herbalists engage in policy advocacy to promote regulations and practices that support sustainability in the herbal industry.

Cultivating a herbal mindset centered on ethics and sustainability is not only a responsibility but also an opportunity to deepen one's connection with nature and contribute to the well-being of the planet. By practicing ethical herbalism, individuals can make a positive impact on plant communities, ecosystems, and the global herbal community. In the subsequent chapters, we will explore specific herbs and their applications, considering the ethical and sustainable aspects of each plant's use in herbal medicine.

Collaboration and Community Engagement

Ethical herbalism often involves collaboration and community engagement. Herbalists recognize the importance of working together to promote sustainability and responsible herbal practices.

Community Herb Gardens: Herbalists may participate in or establish community herb gardens where local residents can learn about, cultivate, and harvest medicinal plants collectively.

Collaborative Conservation: Collaboration with local conservation organizations, botanists, and researchers can lead to the protection and preservation of local plant species.

Transparency and Accountability

Transparency and accountability are key principles of ethical herbalism. Herbalists take responsibility for their actions and decisions and are open about their practices.

Documentation: They maintain records of plant harvests, cultivation practices, and sourcing information, allowing for traceability and accountability.

Consumer Education: Ethical herbalists educate consumers about the importance of transparency in herbal products and encourage them to ask questions about sourcing and sustainability.

Adherence to Regulations

Ethical herbalists are mindful of and adhere to local, national, and international regulations related to the harvesting, cultivation, and trade of medicinal plants.

CITES Compliance: For plants listed under the Convention on International Trade in Endangered Species of Wild Fauna and Flora (CITES), herbalists ensure compliance with CITES regulations to prevent illegal trade and overharvesting.

Permit Requirements: When required, they obtain permits for wildcrafting or cultivating protected or regulated plant species.

Lifelong Learning and Adaptation

Ethical herbalism is a dynamic and evolving practice. Herbalists commit to lifelong learning and adaptation as they gain new insights and information.

Continual Education: They stay updated on developments in herbalism, plant conservation, and sustainable practices through workshops, courses, and engagement with the herbal community.

Adaptation: Ethical herbalists adapt their practices in response to changing ecological conditions and evolving knowledge about plant conservation.

By cultivating a herbal mindset grounded in ethics and sustainability, herbalists contribute to the well-being of the Earth's ecosystems and the longevity of herbal traditions. Ethical herbalism is not a static set of rules but a living practice that evolves in harmony with the natural world. In the chapters that follow, we will explore specific herbs, their therapeutic applications, and how ethical and sustainable considerations are integrated into their use in herbal medicine.

Local and Seasonal Use

Ethical herbalists prioritize the use of locally available and seasonal herbs whenever possible. This approach reduces the carbon footprint associated with transporting herbs long distances and supports local biodiversity.

Local Sourcing: They source herbs from nearby regions or grow them in their own gardens to reduce the environmental impact of transportation.

Seasonal Awareness: Ethical herbalists are attuned to the seasonal availability of herbs and adjust their formulations and remedies accordingly. This not only aligns with ecological rhythms but also enhances the potency of the herbs.

Regenerative Practices

Some herbalists go beyond sustainability and engage in regenerative practices. Regenerative agriculture and wildcrafting aim to restore ecosystems, increase biodiversity, and improve soil health.

Ecosystem Restoration: They actively work to restore damaged ecosystems by planting native species, managing invasive plants, and participating in ecological restoration projects.

Soil Health: Regenerative herbalists prioritize soil health through composting, minimal tillage, and organic farming practices to ensure the long-term vitality of medicinal plants.

Ethical Business Practices

Ethical herbalism extends to business practices. Herbalists who sell herbal products or offer herbal consultations adhere to ethical business principles.

Fair Pricing: They set fair and transparent prices for their products and services, ensuring that herbal medicine remains accessible to diverse communities.

Consumer Education: Ethical herbalists educate consumers about the value of ethically sourced and locally grown herbs, encouraging informed choices.

Advocacy for Plant Conservation

Ethical herbalists often become advocates for plant conservation and sustainable herbal practices, both within the herbal community and on a broader scale.

Public Awareness: They raise public awareness about the importance of plant conservation, habitat protection, and ethical sourcing through workshops, seminars, and educational materials.

Policy Advocacy: Some herbalists actively engage in policy advocacy to influence regulations and policies related to plant conservation and the herbal industry.

Honoring Cultural Traditions

Ethical herbalists honor and respect the cultural traditions and Indigenous knowledge associated with herbal medicine. They seek permission and guidance when working with plants from specific cultural backgrounds.

Cultural Sensitivity: Ethical herbalism acknowledges the potential for cultural appropriation and takes steps to ensure that traditional knowledge and practices are treated with respect and reverence.

2. Understanding Diseases: How Herbs Provide Natural Relief

Chapter 6: The Human Body and Its Ailments

To effectively apply herbal medicine, it's essential to have a foundational understanding of the human body and the various ailments that can affect it. This knowledge provides a framework for selecting the right herbs and treatments to address specific health issues. In this chapter, we'll explore the human body's major systems and common ailments, offering insights into how herbal medicine can be employed for holistic healing.

1. The Circulatory System

The circulatory system, consisting of the heart, blood vessels, and blood, plays a vital role in transporting oxygen, nutrients, and hormones throughout the body. Ailments related to this system include hypertension (high blood pressure), atherosclerosis (hardening of the arteries), and varicose veins.

Herbal Approach: Herbalists use herbs like Hawthorn (Crataegus spp.) to support cardiovascular health by improving blood circulation and regulating blood pressure. Ginger (Zingiber officinale) and Ginkgo biloba are also employed to enhance circulation.

2. The Digestive System

The digestive system encompasses the mouth, esophagus, stomach, intestines, and associated organs. Common digestive ailments include indigestion, acid reflux, irritable bowel syndrome (IBS), and constipation.

Herbal Approach: Herbal remedies like Peppermint (Mentha × piperita) and Ginger (Zingiber officinale) are used to soothe digestive discomfort and relieve symptoms of indigestion. Aloe Vera (Aloe barbadensis) may be employed for its laxative effect to alleviate constipation.

3. The Respiratory System

The respiratory system includes the lungs, bronchi, and trachea, responsible for breathing and oxygen exchange. Ailments here encompass asthma, bronchitis, common colds, and allergies.

Herbal Approach: Herbs such as Echinacea (Echinacea purpurea) and Elderberry (Sambucus nigra) are used to strengthen the immune system and prevent respiratory infections. Mullein (Verbascum thapsus) and Thyme (Thymus vulgaris) can help alleviate symptoms of bronchitis and congestion.

4. The Nervous System

The nervous system, consisting of the central nervous system (brain and spinal cord) and peripheral nervous system, regulates bodily functions and allows us to respond to stimuli. Ailments here include anxiety, depression, insomnia, and neuralgia.

Herbal Approach: Herbal medicine offers calming remedies like Valerian (Valeriana officinalis) and Chamomile (Matricaria chamomilla) to ease anxiety and promote sleep. St. John's Wort (Hypericum perforatum) is used to address mild to moderate depression.

5. The Musculoskeletal System

The musculoskeletal system comprises muscles, bones, joints, and connective tissues. Common ailments involve arthritis, muscle pain, sprains, and fractures.

Herbal Approach: Herbs like Devil's Claw (Harpagophytum procumbens) and Turmeric (Curcuma longa) are used for their anti-inflammatory properties to alleviate pain associated with arthritis. Arnica (Arnica montana) is employed topically for muscle pain and bruises.

6. The Immune System

The immune system defends the body against infections and diseases. Ailments include frequent infections, autoimmune disorders, and weakened immunity.

Herbal Approach: Immune-boosting herbs like Astragalus (Astragalus membranaceus) and Echinacea (Echinacea purpurea) are used to strengthen the immune response. Medicinal mushrooms such as Reishi (Ganoderma lucidum) also support immune function.

7. The Reproductive System

The reproductive system encompasses the male and female reproductive organs. Ailments involve menstrual irregularities, infertility, erectile dysfunction, and menopause-related symptoms.

Herbal Approach: Herbs like Chaste Tree Berry (Vitex agnus-castus) can help regulate menstrual cycles and relieve PMS symptoms in women. Maca (Lepidium meyenii) is known for its potential to improve fertility, while Horny Goat Weed (Epimedium spp.) is used for erectile dysfunction.

8. The Integumentary System

The integumentary system includes the skin, hair, and nails. Common ailments involve skin conditions like eczema, acne, psoriasis, and fungal infections.

Herbal Approach: Herbs like Calendula (Calendula officinalis) and Lavender (Lavandula angustifolia) are used topically for their soothing and anti-inflammatory effects on the skin. Tea Tree oil (Melaleuca alternifolia) is employed for its antifungal properties.

9. The Endocrine System

The endocrine system consists of glands that produce hormones, regulating various bodily functions such as metabolism, growth, and mood. Ailments in this system include hormonal imbalances, diabetes, thyroid disorders, and adrenal fatigue.

Herbal Approach: Herbs like Ashwagandha (Withania somnifera) and Rhodiola (Rhodiola rosea) are employed to support adrenal health and manage stress-related hormonal imbalances. Cinnamon (Cinnamomum verum) and Fenugreek (Trigonella foenum-graecum) may assist in blood sugar regulation.

10. The Urinary System

The urinary system comprises the kidneys, bladder, and urethra, responsible for filtering waste and maintaining fluid balance. Ailments here include urinary tract infections (UTIs), kidney stones, and bladder issues.

Herbal Approach: Cranberry (Vaccinium macrocarpon) is known for its preventive effect against UTIs. Dandelion (Taraxacum officinale) and Corn Silk (Zea mays) may be used for kidney health and to support urinary function.

11. The Lymphatic System

The lymphatic system is responsible for maintaining fluid balance and supporting the immune system by filtering out toxins and waste. Ailments involve lymphedema, lymphadenitis, and a compromised immune response.

Herbal Approach: Cleavers (Galium aparine) and Red Root (Ceanothus spp.) are used to support lymphatic circulation and drainage. Echinacea (Echinacea purpurea) may be employed to boost immune function.

12. The Gastrointestinal System

The gastrointestinal (GI) system includes the stomach and intestines and is essential for digestion and nutrient absorption. Ailments range from gastritis and food intolerances to inflammatory bowel disease (IBD) and leaky gut syndrome.

Herbal Approach: Herbs like Slippery Elm (Ulmus rubra) and Marshmallow Root (Althaea officinalis) can soothe and heal irritated GI linings. Turmeric (Curcuma longa) and Boswellia (Boswellia serrata) have anti-inflammatory properties beneficial for IBD.

13. The Reproductive System (Male and Female)

The male and female reproductive systems are responsible for reproductive processes. Ailments include fertility issues, sexual dysfunction, polycystic ovary syndrome (PCOS), and endometriosis.

Herbal Approach: For fertility, Tribulus terrestris may be used for men, and Red Clover (Trifolium pratense) for women. Damiana (Turnera diffusa) is employed for sexual dysfunction. Vitex (Vitex agnus-castus) can help regulate hormonal imbalances in women with PCOS.

14. The Metabolic System

The metabolic system encompasses the body's energy production and utilization. Ailments include metabolic syndrome, obesity, and disorders related to metabolic rate.

Herbal Approach: Green Tea (Camellia sinensis) and Garcinia cambogia may support weight management and metabolic health. Cinnamon (Cinnamomum verum) can help regulate blood sugar levels.

15. The Mental and Emotional Health

Mental and emotional health is influenced by various factors, including neurotransmitters and stress hormones. Ailments range from anxiety and depression to stress-related disorders.

Herbal Approach: Adaptogenic herbs like Ashwagandha (Withania somnifera) and Rhodiola (Rhodiola rosea) help the body adapt to stress and support emotional well-being. St. John's Wort (Hypericum perforatum) is used for mild to moderate depression.

16. The Endocannabinoid System

The endocannabinoid system (ECS) is a complex network of receptors and neurotransmitters that play a role in regulating various physiological processes, including pain perception, mood, and immune response. Ailments related to the ECS include chronic pain, anxiety disorders, and autoimmune diseases.

Herbal Approach: Herbs such as Hemp (Cannabis sativa) and CBD-rich strains of Cannabis are increasingly recognized for their potential to interact with the ECS and alleviate symptoms associated with chronic pain, anxiety, and inflammatory conditions.

17. The Vision and Eye Health

The visual system includes the eyes and the complex neural pathways responsible for vision. Ailments encompass conditions like myopia, cataracts, glaucoma, and age-related macular degeneration (AMD).

Herbal Approach: Bilberry (Vaccinium myrtillus) is well-regarded for its potential to support eye health and improve vision, particularly in cases of AMD. Ginkgo biloba may also benefit vision by enhancing blood flow to the eyes.

18. The Ear, Nose, and Throat (ENT)

The ENT system includes the organs responsible for hearing, smelling, and speaking. Ailments here include ear infections, sinusitis, allergies, and sore throats.

Herbal Approach: Herbs like Echinacea (Echinacea purpurea) and Goldenseal (Hydrastis canadensis) are used to boost the immune system and alleviate symptoms of upper respiratory infections. Mullein (Verbascum thapsus) can be helpful for earaches and ear infections.

19. The Endurance and Stamina

Endurance and stamina are vital for physical performance and overall vitality. Ailments involve fatigue, low energy, and conditions like chronic fatigue syndrome.

Herbal Approach: Adaptogenic herbs like Rhodiola (Rhodiola rosea) and Eleuthero (Eleutherococcus senticosus) are used to enhance endurance, combat fatigue, and improve overall stamina. Maca (Lepidium meyenii) may also support energy levels.

20. The Oral Health

Oral health encompasses the mouth, teeth, and gums. Ailments include dental caries, gum disease, and oral infections.

Herbal Approach: Herbs like Myrrh (Commiphora myrrha) and Clove (Syzygium aromaticum) have antimicrobial properties and can be used for oral health, including addressing gum infections and toothaches.

21. The Skin and Hair Health

The skin and hair are visible indicators of overall health and well-being. Ailments encompass skin conditions such as acne, eczema, and hair loss.

Herbal Approach: Topical applications of herbs like Calendula (Calendula officinalis) and Aloe Vera (Aloe barbadensis) can soothe skin irritations and promote healing. Nettle (Urtica dioica) and Saw Palmetto (Serenoa repens) may be used to support hair health.

22. The Environmental Toxins and Detoxification

The body's ability to detoxify and eliminate environmental toxins is crucial for maintaining health. Ailments relate to toxin exposure, including heavy metal toxicity and chemical sensitivities.

Herbal Approach: Herbs such as Milk Thistle (Silybum marianum) and Dandelion (Taraxacum officinale) support liver detoxification. Chlorella and Spirulina are used to assist the body in eliminating heavy metals.

23. The Allergies and Sensitivities

Allergies and sensitivities involve an exaggerated immune response to allergens, leading to symptoms like hay fever, food allergies, and skin reactions.

Herbal Approach: Herbs like Butterbur (Petasites hybridus) and Quercetin have antihistamine and anti-inflammatory properties that can alleviate allergy symptoms. Calendula (Calendula officinalis) and Chamomile (Matricaria chamomilla) may soothe skin reactions.

24. The Autoimmune Disorders

Autoimmune disorders occur when the immune system mistakenly attacks the body's own tissues. Common ailments include rheumatoid arthritis, lupus, and multiple sclerosis.

Herbal Approach: Some herbs, like Turmeric (Curcuma longa) and Ginger (Zingiber officinale), have anti-inflammatory properties that may help manage symptoms of autoimmune conditions. However, treatment should be individualized and supervised by a healthcare professional.

Understanding the intricacies of these additional aspects of the human body and related ailments allows herbalists and individuals to explore the full potential of herbal remedies for holistic health. By selecting the appropriate herbs and treatments based on this knowledge, one can address a wide range of health concerns effectively. In the upcoming chapters, we will delve into specific herbs, their therapeutic applications, and practical guidance for incorporating herbal remedies into daily life, considering the nuances of various health issues.

Chapter 7: How Herbs Interact with the Body

Understanding how herbs interact with the body is fundamental to the practice of herbal medicine. Herbs contain bioactive compounds that can influence various physiological processes and systems. This chapter explores the mechanisms by which herbs exert their effects on the human body, shedding light on the complexities of herbal interactions.

Receptor Binding

Many herbs contain compounds that can bind to specific receptors in the body. Receptors are proteins located on the surface of cells or within cells that are involved in transmitting signals. When an herb's bioactive compounds bind to these receptors, they can either mimic or block the actions of naturally occurring substances in the body.

Example: Cannabinoids found in Cannabis plants bind to cannabinoid receptors in the endocannabinoid system, influencing mood, pain perception, and immune function.

Enzyme Inhibition

Some herbs contain compounds that can inhibit or enhance the activity of enzymes in the body. Enzymes are responsible for facilitating biochemical reactions. By modulating enzyme activity, herbs can affect various metabolic processes.

Example: St. John's Wort contains compounds that can inhibit the activity of cytochrome P450 enzymes, which are involved in drug metabolism. This herb can influence the effectiveness of certain medications.

Anti-Inflammatory Effects

Many herbs possess anti-inflammatory properties. Chronic inflammation is associated with a wide range of health issues, including cardiovascular disease, autoimmune disorders, and cancer. Herbs with anti-inflammatory compounds can help reduce inflammation in the body.

Example: Turmeric contains curcumin, a potent anti-inflammatory compound that can modulate inflammatory pathways and reduce the risk of chronic inflammatory diseases.

Antioxidant Activity

Herbs are rich sources of antioxidants, which help neutralize harmful free radicals in the body. Excessive free radical damage is implicated in aging and various diseases, including cancer and neurodegenerative conditions.

Example: Green tea contains catechins, powerful antioxidants that can protect cells from oxidative stress and reduce the risk of chronic diseases.

Hormonal Modulation

Certain herbs contain compounds that can influence hormone production and regulation. These herbs can be used to balance hormonal levels or alleviate hormonal imbalances.

Example: Chasteberry (Vitex agnus-castus) is known for its ability to modulate hormones and is often used to regulate menstrual cycles and manage symptoms of premenstrual syndrome (PMS).

Immune System Modulation

Herbs can modulate the immune system, either by enhancing or suppressing immune responses. This property can be valuable for conditions involving immune dysfunction.

Example: Echinacea is renowned for its immune-boosting properties and is used to support the body's defense against infections.

Neurotransmitter Influence

Some herbs contain compounds that can affect neurotransmitters, the chemical messengers in the brain and nervous system. These herbs can influence mood, cognition, and behavior.

Example: Ginkgo biloba is believed to enhance cognitive function by improving blood flow to the brain and modulating neurotransmitter activity.

Anti-Microbial Activity

Many herbs have antimicrobial properties, making them effective against bacteria, viruses, fungi, and parasites. They can be used to treat various infections.

Example: Garlic has potent antimicrobial properties and is used to combat bacterial and viral infections.

Relaxation and Stress Reduction

Certain herbs have relaxing and calming effects on the nervous system. They can help reduce stress, anxiety, and promote relaxation.

Example: Valerian is known for its sedative properties and is used to alleviate anxiety and improve sleep quality.

Adaptogenic Properties

Adaptogenic herbs help the body adapt to stressors and maintain balance. They can support overall resilience and well-being.

Example: Ashwagandha is an adaptogen known for its ability to reduce stress and improve energy levels.

Blood Sugar Regulation

Certain herbs can help regulate blood sugar levels, making them valuable for individuals with diabetes or those at risk of developing the condition. These herbs work by enhancing insulin sensitivity or inhibiting the absorption of glucose in the digestive tract.

Example: Cinnamon contains compounds that can improve insulin sensitivity and lower blood sugar levels. It is used as an adjunct therapy for diabetes management.

Diuretic Effects

Diuretic herbs promote increased urine production and can be beneficial for conditions involving excess fluid retention or hypertension. They help the body eliminate excess sodium and water.

Example: Dandelion leaf (Taraxacum officinale) is a diuretic herb that is often used to reduce water retention and support kidney health.

Digestive Aid

Many herbs have digestive properties that can help alleviate symptoms of indigestion, bloating, and gas. These herbs can stimulate digestive enzymes and promote healthy digestion.

Example: Ginger is known for its digestive benefits and is used to relieve nausea, reduce bloating, and improve overall digestion.

Cardiovascular Support

Herbs with cardiovascular benefits can help maintain heart health and reduce the risk of cardiovascular diseases. They often work by reducing blood pressure, improving cholesterol profiles, and enhancing blood vessel function.

Example: Hawthorn (Crataegus spp.) is a well-known herb for cardiovascular support. It can improve heart function, reduce blood pressure, and support overall cardiovascular health.

Anti-Anxiety and Mood Enhancement

Certain herbs have a calming and mood-enhancing effect on the nervous system. They can be valuable for managing anxiety, depression, and mood disorders.

Example: Lemon Balm (Melissa officinalis) has mild sedative properties and is used to reduce anxiety and promote relaxation.

Anti-Allergic Properties

Herbs with anti-allergic properties can help alleviate symptoms of allergies, such as sneezing, congestion, and itchy eyes. They often work by stabilizing mast cells and reducing histamine release.

Example: Butterbur (Petasites hybridus) is used as a natural remedy for seasonal allergies and allergic rhinitis.

Anti-Coagulant Effects

Some herbs possess mild anti-coagulant or blood-thinning properties, which can be beneficial for individuals at risk of blood clots or cardiovascular events.

Example: Ginkgo biloba can improve blood circulation and reduce the risk of blood clots, making it suitable for individuals with poor circulation.

Detoxification Support

Herbs can assist the body's detoxification processes by promoting the elimination of toxins through the liver, kidneys, and digestive system.

Example: Milk Thistle (Silybum marianum) is known for its liver-protective properties and is used to support liver detoxification.

Anti-Aging and Skin Health

Certain herbs contain antioxidants and compounds that can promote skin health, reduce signs of aging, and protect the skin from environmental damage.

Example: Green tea extract is used in skincare products for its antioxidant properties, which can help reduce skin aging and improve complexion.

Hormone Regulation

Herbs can influence hormonal balance by either mimicking or modulating the effects of hormones in the body. They can be valuable for conditions involving hormonal imbalances.

Example: Black Cohosh (Actaea racemosa) is used to alleviate symptoms of menopause by modulating estrogen levels.

Understanding these diverse mechanisms of herbal action allows herbalists and individuals to select the most appropriate herbs for specific health concerns. It also highlights the potential for herbal medicine to complement conventional treatments and promote holistic health. In the subsequent chapters, we will delve into specific herbs, their therapeutic applications, and practical guidance for using them effectively in various health contexts.

Antispasmodic and Muscle Relaxant Properties

Certain herbs have antispasmodic properties that can help relieve muscle spasms and tension. These herbs are valuable for conditions involving muscle cramps and discomfort.

Example: Cramp bark (Viburnum opulus) is used to alleviate uterine and muscle cramps, making it beneficial for menstrual pain and muscle tension.

Antiviral Activity

Herbs with antiviral properties can help the body combat viral infections. They often work by inhibiting viral replication or strengthening the immune response against viruses.

Example: Elderberry (Sambucus nigra) is known for its antiviral effects and is used to reduce the severity and duration of cold and flu symptoms.

Anti-Ulcer and Gastric Protection

Some herbs can protect the stomach lining and reduce the risk of gastric ulcers. They often have soothing and anti-inflammatory properties for the digestive tract.

Example: Licorice root (Glycyrrhiza glabra) contains compounds that can help heal gastric ulcers and relieve symptoms of heartburn and gastritis.

Anti-Parasitic Effects

Certain herbs possess anti-parasitic properties and can be used to combat parasitic infections in the digestive system.

Example: Wormwood (Artemisia absinthium) is traditionally used to treat intestinal parasites, such as roundworms and pinworms.

Memory Enhancement and Cognitive Support

Herbs can enhance cognitive function and support memory retention. They often work by improving blood flow to the brain and protecting brain cells.

Example: Bacopa monnieri is an herb known for its cognitive-enhancing effects and is used to support memory and learning.

Anti-Inflammatory Effects on Joints

In addition to their general anti-inflammatory properties, some herbs specifically target joint inflammation, making them useful for conditions like arthritis.

Example: Boswellia (Boswellia serrata) is known for its anti-inflammatory effects on joints and is used to alleviate symptoms of osteoarthritis and rheumatoid arthritis.

Antioxidant for Eye Health

Certain herbs contain antioxidants that are beneficial for eye health. They can protect the eyes from oxidative stress and age-related conditions like macular degeneration.

Example: Bilberry (Vaccinium myrtillus) is rich in antioxidants and is used to support eye health and improve vision.

Immune-Modulating Effects

Herbs with immune-modulating effects can help balance immune responses, making them valuable for autoimmune disorders where the immune system is overactive.

Example: Astragalus (Astragalus membranaceus) is used to support immune function and balance the immune response in autoimmune conditions.

Relaxation of Smooth Muscles

Some herbs have a relaxing effect on smooth muscles in the body, which can be valuable for conditions involving muscle spasms or tension in the gastrointestinal or respiratory systems.

Example: Lobelia (Lobelia inflata) is known for its muscle-relaxing properties and can be used for respiratory conditions involving bronchospasms.

Understanding these diverse mechanisms of herbal action allows herbalists and individuals to select the most appropriate herbs for specific health concerns. It also highlights the potential for herbal medicine to complement conventional treatments and promote holistic health. In the subsequent chapters, we will delve into specific herbs, their therapeutic applications, and practical guidance for using them effectively in various health contexts.

Chapter 8: Herbal Support for Common Illnesses

Herbal medicine offers a natural and holistic approach to managing a wide range of common illnesses. In this chapter, we will explore how specific herbs can be used to provide support and relief for various health conditions. While herbs can be a valuable addition to a wellness routine, it's essential to consult with a qualified herbalist or healthcare professional, especially for chronic or serious health issues.

1. Respiratory Infections

Respiratory infections, such as the common cold and flu, are prevalent health concerns. Herbs can provide relief from symptoms and support the body's immune response.

Herbal Support:

Echinacea: This immune-boosting herb can help shorten the duration and severity of colds and flu.

Elderberry: Known for its antiviral properties, elderberry can reduce symptoms and speed up recovery.

Peppermint and Thyme: These herbs can relieve congestion, soothe sore throats, and ease breathing difficulties.

2. Digestive Disorders

Digestive disorders like indigestion, bloating, and irritable bowel syndrome (IBS) can be uncomfortable. Herbs can help soothe digestive discomfort.

Herbal Support:

Ginger: An excellent digestive aid, ginger can alleviate nausea, indigestion, and gas.

Peppermint: This herb relaxes the gastrointestinal muscles, reducing spasms and discomfort.

Chamomile: Chamomile tea can calm an upset stomach and ease digestive distress.

3. Stress and Anxiety

Stress and anxiety can impact mental and physical health. Herbal remedies can promote relaxation and reduce stress.

Herbal Support:

Valerian: Valerian root has sedative properties and can help with anxiety and sleep disorders.

Passionflower: This herb can induce relaxation and alleviate symptoms of anxiety.

Lemon Balm: Lemon balm is calming and can reduce stress and anxiety.

4. Sleep Disturbances

Sleep is essential for overall well-being, and herbal remedies can aid in achieving restful sleep.

Herbal Support:

Lavender: Lavender essential oil or tea can promote relaxation and improve sleep quality.

Valerian: Valerian root is commonly used to alleviate insomnia and promote restful sleep.

Chamomile: Chamomile tea can have a mild sedative effect and improve sleep.

5. Skin Conditions

Skin conditions like eczema, acne, and psoriasis can be uncomfortable and affect self-esteem. Certain herbs have soothing properties for the skin.

Herbal Support:

Calendula: Calendula salve or cream can soothe irritated skin and promote healing.

Aloe Vera: Aloe gel can provide relief for sunburn and minor skin irritations.

Tea Tree Oil: Tea tree oil has antimicrobial properties and can be used for acne and fungal skin infections.

6. Allergies

Allergies can result in sneezing, congestion, and itchy eyes. Herbs with anti-allergic properties can provide relief.

Herbal Support:

Butterbur: Butterbur supplements can reduce symptoms of seasonal allergies.

Quercetin: This flavonoid found in foods like onions and apples has antihistamine properties.

Nettle: Nettle tea or supplements can alleviate hay fever symptoms.

7. Pain and Inflammation

Chronic pain and inflammation can be debilitating. Herbal remedies can offer relief and support healing.

Herbal Support:

Turmeric: Turmeric's curcumin compound has potent anti-inflammatory properties.

Willow Bark: Willow bark contains salicin, a natural pain reliever similar to aspirin.

Arnica: Arnica gel or cream can reduce pain and inflammation from injuries.

8. Menstrual Discomfort

Menstrual cramps and PMS symptoms can disrupt daily life. Herbal remedies can help regulate the menstrual cycle and alleviate discomfort.

Herbal Support:

Chaste Tree Berry: Chaste tree berry can help regulate hormonal imbalances and ease PMS symptoms.

Dong Quai: This herb is used in Traditional Chinese Medicine to alleviate menstrual pain and support hormonal balance.

Ginger: Ginger tea can relieve menstrual cramps and reduce pain.

9. Joint and Muscle Pain

Joint pain and muscle soreness are common issues, especially as we age or engage in physical activities. Herbal remedies can provide relief and reduce inflammation.

Herbal Support:

Devil's Claw: Devil's Claw is known for its anti-inflammatory properties and can help with osteoarthritis and muscle pain.

Boswellia: Boswellia extract can reduce joint inflammation and improve mobility in conditions like rheumatoid arthritis.

Arnica: Arnica cream or oil is used topically to alleviate muscle pain, stiffness, and bruising.

10. Urinary Tract Infections (UTIs)

UTIs can be painful and require prompt treatment. Certain herbs can help alleviate symptoms and support urinary tract health.

Herbal Support:

Cranberry: Cranberry juice or supplements can prevent UTIs by preventing bacteria from adhering to the urinary tract lining.

Dandelion: Dandelion tea can promote urine production and help flush out bacteria from the urinary tract.

Uva Ursi: Uva ursi has antimicrobial properties and can be used as a natural remedy for UTIs.

11. High Blood Pressure (Hypertension)

High blood pressure is a risk factor for heart disease and stroke. Herbal remedies can complement lifestyle changes to manage blood pressure.

Herbal Support:

Hawthorn: Hawthorn extracts can dilate blood vessels and improve blood flow, helping to lower blood pressure.

Garlic: Garlic supplements can have a mild blood pressure-lowering effect.

Olive Leaf: Olive leaf extract may reduce blood pressure by relaxing blood vessels.

12. Immune System Boost

Strengthening the immune system is essential for overall health, especially during cold and flu seasons. Certain herbs can enhance immune function.

Herbal Support:

Astragalus: Astragalus root is an immune-boosting herb that can enhance the body's defenses against infections.

Reishi Mushroom: Reishi is a medicinal mushroom known for its immune-modulating properties.

Echinacea: Echinacea supplements can stimulate the immune system and reduce the severity of colds and respiratory infections.

13. Headaches and Migraines

Headaches and migraines can be debilitating. Herbal remedies can help alleviate pain and reduce the frequency of attacks.

Herbal Support:

Feverfew: Feverfew supplements may reduce the frequency and severity of migraines.

Peppermint: Peppermint oil applied topically or inhaled can provide relief from tension headaches.

Butterbur: Butterbur extracts have been shown to be effective in preventing migraines.

14. Seasonal Affective Disorder (SAD)

Seasonal affective disorder is a type of depression that occurs at specific times of the year, typically in the winter months. Herbal remedies can help improve mood and alleviate symptoms.

Herbal Support:

St. John's Wort: St. John's Wort is known for its antidepressant effects and can be used to manage mild to moderate depression, including SAD.

Rhodiola: Rhodiola is an adaptogen that can help increase energy levels and reduce fatigue associated with SAD.

Saffron: Saffron supplements may improve mood and reduce symptoms of depression.

15. Memory and Cognitive Function

Memory decline and cognitive impairment are concerns as we age. Certain herbs can support brain health and cognitive function.

Herbal Support:

Ginkgo Biloba: Ginkgo biloba extracts can enhance memory, concentration, and blood flow to the brain.

Bacopa Monnieri: Bacopa is known for its cognitive-enhancing properties and can improve memory and learning.

Gotu Kola: Gotu kola is used to enhance cognitive function and improve mental clarity.

Herbal medicine provides a vast array of remedies for addressing common health issues. When considering herbal support for specific conditions, it's crucial to consult with a qualified herbalist or healthcare professional to ensure the safety and effectiveness of herbal treatments. Integrating herbal remedies with conventional healthcare can lead to a holistic approach to managing health and well-being.

16. Menopause Symptoms

Menopause can bring about a range of uncomfortable symptoms, including hot flashes, mood swings, and sleep disturbances. Herbal remedies can help alleviate these challenges.

Herbal Support:

Black Cohosh: Black cohosh is known for its ability to reduce hot flashes and other menopause-related symptoms.

Red Clover: Red clover supplements contain compounds called isoflavones, which can help with menopausal symptoms.

Dong Quai: Dong quai is used in Traditional Chinese Medicine to balance hormones and relieve menopausal discomfort.

17. Respiratory Conditions (Asthma, Bronchitis)

Chronic respiratory conditions like asthma and bronchitis can be managed with the help of herbal remedies that support lung health and reduce inflammation.

Herbal Support:

Licorice Root: Licorice root has soothing properties for the respiratory tract and can ease coughs and inflammation.

Mullein: Mullein tea is known for its ability to soothe respiratory discomfort and ease breathing.

Osha Root: Osha root is used in Native American herbal medicine to alleviate respiratory conditions.

18. Joint Health and Osteoarthritis

Maintaining joint health is crucial for mobility and quality of life. Herbal remedies can provide support and reduce inflammation in conditions like osteoarthritis.

Herbal Support:

Turmeric: Turmeric's anti-inflammatory compound, curcumin, can help reduce joint pain and stiffness.

Ginger: Ginger supplements or teas can alleviate symptoms of osteoarthritis by reducing inflammation.

Boswellia: Boswellia extracts can improve joint function and reduce pain in osteoarthritis.

19. High Cholesterol

High cholesterol levels are a risk factor for heart disease. Herbal remedies can be used in conjunction with dietary and lifestyle changes to manage cholesterol levels.

Herbal Support:

Garlic: Garlic supplements may help lower LDL cholesterol levels and improve overall heart health.

Artichoke Leaf: Artichoke leaf extracts can have a cholesterol-lowering effect and support liver health.

Psyllium: Psyllium husk supplements can help reduce cholesterol levels by binding to dietary cholesterol in the digestive tract.

20. Gastroesophageal Reflux Disease (GERD)

GERD is a digestive disorder characterized by acid reflux and heartburn. Herbal remedies can help manage symptoms and promote digestive health.

Herbal Support:

Slippery Elm: Slippery elm supplements or tea can soothe the esophagus and reduce the discomfort of acid reflux.

Marshmallow Root: Marshmallow root has mucilaginous properties that can alleviate irritation in the esophagus.

Ginger: Ginger can help reduce symptoms of GERD by promoting healthy digestion and reducing inflammation.

Chapter 9: Chronic Conditions and Herbal Interventions

Chronic conditions are long-term health issues that require ongoing management. While herbal interventions are not a replacement for medical treatment, they can complement conventional therapies and provide support for individuals living with chronic illnesses. In this chapter, we explore how specific herbs can be used as part of an integrative approach to managing chronic conditions. It's crucial to work with healthcare professionals or herbalists when incorporating herbs into a treatment plan for chronic conditions.

Diabetes

Diabetes is a chronic condition characterized by high blood sugar levels. Herbal remedies can help manage blood sugar levels and support overall health for individuals with diabetes.

Herbal Interventions:

Cinnamon: Cinnamon supplements or tea can improve insulin sensitivity and help regulate blood sugar levels.

Gymnema: Gymnema sylvestre supplements may reduce sugar cravings and help lower blood sugar.

Fenugreek: Fenugreek seeds can be beneficial for diabetes management by improving glucose tolerance.

Hypothyroidism

Hypothyroidism occurs when the thyroid gland doesn't produce enough thyroid hormones. Herbal interventions can help support thyroid function.

Herbal Interventions:

Ashwagandha: Ashwagandha supplements can help balance thyroid hormones and support overall thyroid health.

Bladderwrack: Bladderwrack contains iodine, which is essential for thyroid function and can be used as a natural thyroid support.

Selenium: Selenium supplements can help support the conversion of thyroid hormones and improve thyroid function.

Hypertension (High Blood Pressure)

High blood pressure is a common chronic condition that increases the risk of heart disease. Herbal interventions can complement lifestyle changes and medications.

Herbal Interventions:

Hawthorn: Hawthorn extracts can dilate blood vessels and help lower blood pressure.

Olive Leaf: Olive leaf extract has been shown to reduce blood pressure by relaxing blood vessels.

Celery Seed: Celery seed supplements can help lower blood pressure due to their diuretic effect.

Inflammatory Bowel Disease (IBD)

Inflammatory bowel diseases like Crohn's disease and ulcerative colitis are chronic conditions that affect the digestive tract. Herbal interventions can help manage symptoms and reduce inflammation.

Herbal Interventions:

Aloe Vera: Aloe vera gel can soothe the digestive tract and reduce inflammation in individuals with IBD.

Turmeric: Turmeric's anti-inflammatory properties can help alleviate symptoms and reduce inflammation.

Marshmallow Root: Marshmallow root has mucilaginous properties that can soothe the intestinal lining.

Chronic Pain

Chronic pain conditions like fibromyalgia and neuropathy can significantly impact quality of life. Herbal interventions can offer pain relief and improve overall well-being.

Herbal Interventions:

Kratom: Kratom leaves contain alkaloids that can provide pain relief and improve mood in individuals with chronic pain.

White Willow Bark: White willow bark supplements contain salicin, a natural pain reliever similar to aspirin.

Corydalis Yanhusuo: Corydalis yanhusuo is used in Traditional Chinese Medicine for pain relief.

Autoimmune Diseases

Autoimmune diseases involve the immune system mistakenly attacking the body's own tissues. Herbal interventions can help modulate the immune response and reduce symptoms.

Herbal Interventions:

Turmeric: Turmeric's curcumin compound has anti-inflammatory properties that may help manage symptoms of autoimmune diseases.

Astragalus: Astragalus root can help balance immune function and reduce inflammation in autoimmune conditions.

Licorice Root: Licorice root can support adrenal function and reduce inflammation in autoimmune diseases.

Chronic Fatigue Syndrome (CFS)

CFS is characterized by persistent, unexplained fatigue. Herbal interventions can help improve energy levels and overall well-being.

Herbal Interventions:

Rhodiola: Rhodiola supplements can combat fatigue, enhance energy levels, and improve mental clarity.

Ashwagandha: Ashwagandha is an adaptogen that can help reduce stress-related fatigue.

Panax Ginseng: Panax ginseng can improve physical and mental performance in individuals with CFS.

Chronic Skin Conditions (Psoriasis, Eczema)

Chronic skin conditions can be uncomfortable and affect self-esteem. Herbal interventions can soothe skin and reduce inflammation.

Herbal Interventions:

Chickweed: Chickweed salves or creams can soothe itching and inflammation in psoriasis and eczema.

Burdock Root: Burdock root supplements can help purify the blood and improve skin health.

Calendula: Calendula salves or oils can promote healing and reduce inflammation in chronic skin conditions.

Chronic Kidney Disease (CKD)

Chronic kidney disease is a long-term condition that affects the kidneys' ability to filter blood effectively. Herbal interventions can be used to support kidney function and manage related symptoms.

Herbal Interventions:

Nettle: Nettle leaf tea or supplements can help improve kidney function and reduce fluid retention.

Dandelion: Dandelion root is a diuretic herb that can support kidney health and promote the elimination of waste.

Cordyceps: Cordyceps supplements are known for their potential to enhance kidney function and overall vitality.

Chronic Respiratory Conditions (COPD)

Chronic obstructive pulmonary disease (COPD) is a progressive lung disease that can cause breathing difficulties. Herbal interventions can assist in managing symptoms and improving lung health.

Herbal Interventions:

Lobelia: Lobelia can relax bronchial passages and improve airflow, making it beneficial for COPD symptoms.

Mullein: Mullein is known for its ability to soothe coughing and reduce inflammation in the respiratory tract.

Elecampane: Elecampane root can help alleviate symptoms of bronchitis and support respiratory health.

Chronic Anxiety and Depression

Chronic anxiety and depression can significantly impact one's mental and emotional well-being. Herbal interventions can be used alongside psychotherapy and other treatments to manage symptoms.

Herbal Interventions:

St. John's Wort: St. John's Wort is a well-known herbal remedy for mild to moderate depression and anxiety.

Lavender: Lavender essential oil or supplements can help reduce symptoms of anxiety and promote relaxation.

Passionflower: Passionflower can induce a calming effect and ease symptoms of anxiety and nervousness.

Chronic Neurological Conditions (Parkinson's, Alzheimer's)

Chronic neurological conditions like Parkinson's and Alzheimer's disease require comprehensive care. Herbal interventions can complement medical treatments and support cognitive function.

Herbal Interventions:

Ginkgo Biloba: Ginkgo biloba extracts can improve cognitive function and memory in individuals with Alzheimer's disease.

Huperzine A: Huperzine A is a natural cholinesterase inhibitor that may help improve memory in Alzheimer's patients.

Mucuna Pruriens: Mucuna pruriens contains levodopa, a precursor to dopamine, and may assist in managing Parkinson's disease symptoms.

Chronic Insomnia

Chronic insomnia can have a significant impact on overall health and quality of life. Herbal interventions can promote better sleep and relaxation.

Herbal Interventions:

Valerian: Valerian root can improve sleep quality and reduce the time it takes to fall asleep.

Melatonin: Melatonin supplements can help regulate sleep-wake cycles and improve sleep patterns.

Chamomile: Chamomile tea can induce relaxation and promote better sleep.

Chronic Digestive Disorders (Crohn's Disease, IBS)

Chronic digestive disorders like Crohn's disease and irritable bowel syndrome (IBS) require ongoing management. Herbal interventions can help alleviate symptoms and support gastrointestinal health.

Herbal Interventions:

Peppermint: Peppermint oil capsules can relieve symptoms of IBS, including abdominal pain and bloating.

Slippery Elm: Slippery elm supplements can soothe the gastrointestinal lining and reduce irritation.

Ginger: Ginger can alleviate nausea and digestive discomfort in individuals with chronic digestive disorders.

Chronic Cardiovascular Conditions (Heart Disease)

Chronic cardiovascular conditions, such as heart disease, require comprehensive care to manage risk factors and improve heart health.

Herbal Interventions:

Garlic: Garlic supplements may help lower LDL cholesterol levels and support overall cardiovascular health.

Cayenne Pepper: Cayenne pepper can improve blood circulation and support heart function.

Motherwort: Motherwort can help reduce heart palpitations and anxiety associated with heart conditions.

Chronic Skin Conditions (Rosacea, Acne)

Skin conditions like rosacea and acne can persist over time and affect one's appearance and self-esteem. Herbal interventions can help manage symptoms and promote skin health.

Herbal Interventions:

Chamomile: Chamomile's anti-inflammatory properties can soothe skin irritation and reduce redness in rosacea.

Tea Tree Oil: Tea tree oil has antimicrobial properties and can be used to manage acne and reduce breakouts.

Licorice Root: Licorice root extracts can help calm redness and inflammation in both rosacea and acne.

Chronic Liver Conditions (Hepatitis, Cirrhosis)

Chronic liver conditions, such as hepatitis and cirrhosis, require ongoing care to support liver function and minimize damage.

Herbal Interventions:

Milk Thistle: Milk thistle is known for its liver-protective properties and can assist in managing liver conditions.

Dandelion: Dandelion root can promote liver detoxification and improve liver function.

Burdock Root: Burdock root supplements can help purify the blood and support liver health.

Chronic Respiratory Conditions (Asthma, Bronchitis)

Chronic respiratory conditions like asthma and chronic bronchitis require consistent management to control symptoms and improve lung function.

Herbal Interventions:

Boswellia: Boswellia extracts can help reduce inflammation in the airways and improve lung function.

Elecampane: Elecampane root can alleviate bronchial congestion and reduce coughing in chronic bronchitis.

Mullein: Mullein is known for its ability to soothe respiratory discomfort and improve lung health.

Chronic Urinary Tract Conditions (Interstitial Cystitis, Recurrent UTIs)

Chronic urinary tract conditions, such as interstitial cystitis and recurrent urinary tract infections (UTIs), require ongoing support for bladder and urinary health.

Herbal Interventions:

Cranberry: Cranberry supplements can help prevent recurrent UTIs by preventing bacteria from adhering to the urinary tract.

Marshmallow Root: Marshmallow root can soothe the bladder lining and alleviate symptoms of interstitial cystitis.

Uva Ursi: Uva ursi has antimicrobial properties and can be used as a natural remedy for chronic UTIs.

Chronic Fatigue Syndrome (CFS)

Chronic fatigue syndrome is characterized by persistent, unexplained fatigue that can severely impact daily life. Herbal interventions can help improve energy levels and overall well-being.

Herbal Interventions:

Rhodiola: Rhodiola supplements can combat fatigue, enhance energy levels, and improve mental clarity in individuals with CFS.

Ashwagandha: Ashwagandha is an adaptogen that can help reduce stress-related fatigue and support adrenal function.

Licorice Root: Licorice root can support adrenal health and improve energy levels in individuals with CFS.

Chapter 10: Prevention: Building Immunity with Herbs

Prevention is a cornerstone of holistic health, and herbs can play a significant role in supporting the immune system and preventing illness. In this chapter, we'll explore how herbs can be used proactively to boost immunity and enhance overall well-being.

Herbal Immune Tonics

Herbal immune tonics are preparations that can help strengthen the immune system over time. They often contain a combination of immune-boosting herbs and are taken regularly to build resilience against infections.

Examples:

Echinacea: Echinacea is a well-known immune-boosting herb that can be taken as a tonic to enhance immune function.

Astragalus: Astragalus root is used as a tonic in Traditional Chinese Medicine to support immune health.

Reishi Mushroom: Reishi is an adaptogenic mushroom that can strengthen the immune system when consumed regularly.

Adaptogenic Herbs

Adaptogenic herbs help the body adapt to stressors, including those that can weaken the immune system. By reducing the impact of stress on the body, these herbs indirectly support immunity.

Examples:

Ashwagandha: Ashwagandha is an adaptogenic herb that can help reduce stress and improve immune function.

Rhodiola: Rhodiola is known for its stress-reducing properties, which can indirectly enhance immunity.

Holy Basil (Tulsi): Holy basil is an adaptogen that can improve the body's resilience to stressors, including infections.

Antioxidant-Rich Herbs

Antioxidants help protect cells from oxidative stress and support overall health. Herbs rich in antioxidants can help reduce inflammation and strengthen the immune system.

Examples:

Turmeric: Turmeric contains curcumin, a potent antioxidant with anti-inflammatory properties.

Ginger: Ginger is rich in antioxidants and can help combat inflammation.

Green Tea: Green tea is abundant in antioxidants called catechins, which can boost immune function.

Elderberry for Immune Support

Elderberry is a specific herb worth highlighting for its immune-boosting properties. Elderberry syrup or supplements are commonly used during the cold and flu season to reduce the severity and duration of illnesses.

Elderberry: Elderberry has antiviral properties that can help the body fight off respiratory infections. It's a popular choice for immune support.

Immunomodulating Herbs

Immunomodulating herbs help regulate the immune system, making them valuable for autoimmune conditions where the immune system is overactive or for supporting immune function when it's compromised.

Examples:

Astragalus: Astragalus can balance immune function and is used in cases of both immune deficiency and autoimmunity.

Licorice Root: Licorice root has immunomodulating effects and can be used to support the immune system's balance.

Herbs for Respiratory Health

Maintaining healthy respiratory function is crucial for preventing respiratory infections. Certain herbs can support lung health and reduce the risk of infections.

Examples:

Thyme: Thyme has antimicrobial properties and can support respiratory health.

Osha Root: Osha root is used traditionally to improve lung function and prevent respiratory infections.

Mullein: Mullein is known for its soothing effect on the respiratory tract and can help prevent infections.

Gut Health and Immunity

A healthy gut microbiome is closely linked to a robust immune system. Probiotic-rich herbs and those that support digestive health can indirectly enhance immunity.

Examples:

Ginger: Ginger supports digestion and can promote a healthy gut microbiome.

Chamomile: Chamomile can soothe digestive discomfort and promote gut health.

Peppermint: Peppermint aids digestion and can support a balanced gut microbiome.

Lifestyle Factors and Herbal Support

In addition to herbal interventions, lifestyle factors like a balanced diet, regular exercise, quality sleep, and stress management are crucial for a strong immune system. Herbs can complement these efforts by providing additional support.

Herbal Support for Stress Management

Stress is a significant factor that can weaken the immune system. Chronic stress can lead to immune dysfunction, making the body more susceptible to infections. Herbal remedies that help manage stress can indirectly enhance immunity by reducing the negative impact of stress on the body.

Examples:

Lemon Balm: Lemon balm is a calming herb that can reduce stress and anxiety, promoting a more resilient immune system.

Passionflower: Passionflower is known for its ability to induce relaxation and alleviate symptoms of stress, indirectly supporting immunity.

Valerian: Valerian root has sedative properties that can improve sleep quality, reducing the body's stress response.

Herbal Preparations for Immune Support

Herbs can be consumed in various forms to support immunity. Besides teas and tonics, herbal preparations such as tinctures, capsules, and herbal soups can provide a convenient way to incorporate immune-boosting herbs into your daily routine.

Examples:

Echinacea Tincture: Echinacea tinctures are concentrated extracts that can be taken daily or during the onset of illness to strengthen the immune response.

Astragalus Capsules: Astragalus capsules provide a convenient way to incorporate this immune-supporting herb into your daily regimen.

Garlic Soup: Garlic is well-known for its immune-boosting properties. Preparing garlic soup with immune-supporting herbs like thyme and ginger can be a delicious and nutritious way to enhance immunity.

Seasonal Herbal Strategies

The immune system's needs may vary with the seasons and environmental factors. Herbalists often recommend different herbs and strategies for each season to adapt to changing immune challenges.

Examples:

Elderberry Syrup for Winter: Elderberry syrup is a popular choice during the winter months to ward off colds and flu.

Nettle Tea for Spring: Nettle tea is often consumed in spring to support allergy-prone individuals by reducing histamine responses.

Peppermint and Chamomile for Summer: Peppermint and chamomile teas can help with digestion and relaxation during the summer when stressors may vary.

Herbal Education and Consultation

To make the most of herbal prevention and immune support, it's essential to seek guidance from qualified herbalists or healthcare professionals. They can provide personalized recommendations tailored to your specific needs and health goals, ensuring that the chosen herbs are safe and effective for you.

Incorporating Culinary Herbs for Immune Health

Many culinary herbs not only add flavor to your dishes but also have immune-boosting properties. Incorporating these herbs into your daily meals can be a delicious way to support your immune system.

Examples:

Rosemary: Rosemary not only adds a savory flavor to dishes but also contains antioxidants that can boost immunity.

Thyme: Thyme is rich in vitamins and can enhance the immune system while adding depth to your cooking.

Oregano: Oregano is known for its antiviral and antibacterial properties, making it a valuable addition to meals during cold and flu season.

Herbal Teas for Immune Resilience

Herbal teas are a soothing way to enjoy the benefits of immune-boosting herbs. Different herbal teas can be chosen based on your preferences and specific immune needs.

Examples:

Ginger and Lemon Tea: Ginger and lemon tea can provide warmth and comfort while boosting the immune system with their antioxidants and vitamin C content.

Echinacea and Goldenseal Tea: This tea combination can be used during the early stages of illness to support the body's defense mechanisms.

Chamomile and Lavender Tea: Chamomile and lavender tea can promote relaxation and stress reduction, indirectly supporting immunity.

Herbal Gardening for Immunity

Growing your own medicinal herbs at home can be a fulfilling way to ensure a fresh and accessible supply of immune-boosting plants. It also connects you with nature and the healing power of plants.

Examples:

Echinacea: Echinacea is a hardy perennial that can thrive in many climates and is excellent for immune support.

Lemon Balm: Lemon balm is easy to grow and can be used for stress reduction and mild immune support.

Calendula: Calendula flowers can be harvested and dried to make soothing teas and salves for skin health and immune support.

Herbal Safety and Allergies

While herbs offer numerous health benefits, it's important to be aware of potential allergies and interactions with medications. Consult with a healthcare professional or herbalist, especially if you have known allergies or are taking medications, to ensure the herbs you choose are safe for you.

3. The Art of Crafting Herbal Remedies: A Step-by-Step Guide

Chapter 11: Essential Tools and Ingredients

To practice herbal medicine effectively, it's crucial to have the right tools and ingredients at your disposal. This chapter explores the essential equipment, supplies, and ingredients that are fundamental to herbal medicine preparation and application.

Mortar and Pestle

A mortar and pestle are invaluable tools for grinding and crushing herbs, roots, and other plant materials. This manual method allows you to prepare herbs for various uses, such as making teas, poultices, or tinctures.

Herb Grinder

An herb grinder is a practical alternative to a mortar and pestle, especially for grinding dried herbs quickly and efficiently. It's essential for preparing herbs for capsules, tinctures, or herbal blends.

Herb Infusion Tools

Teapot or Teakettle: For making herbal infusions (teas), a teapot or teakettle with an infuser or built-in strainer is helpful.

Tea Strainer or Infuser Basket: These tools help strain loose herb leaves and flowers when making herbal teas.

Tincture Bottles

Tinctures are concentrated herbal extracts preserved in alcohol or glycerin. Tincture bottles with droppers or pipettes allow for precise dosing and storage of tinctured herbs.

Drying Racks

Drying racks or screens are essential for air-drying fresh herbs or roots. Proper drying prevents mold and ensures the herbs retain their potency.

Herbal Storage Containers

Storing dried herbs correctly is crucial to maintain their freshness and potency. Glass jars with airtight lids are ideal for this purpose. Label each container with the herb's name and date of harvest or purchase.

Carrier Oils

Carrier oils, such as olive oil, coconut oil, or almond oil, are used to make herbal infused oils for topical applications like massages, salves, and skin treatments.

Beeswax

Beeswax is often used in herbal salve recipes to provide a solid texture and help maintain the salve's consistency.

Double Boiler

A double boiler is essential for gentle heating and melting of ingredients when making herbal salves, balms, or ointments.

Cheesecloth or Muslin Bags

Cheesecloth or muslin bags are used for straining herbal infusions, creating herbal sachets, or making poultices.

Glass Measuring Cups and Spoons

Accurate measurements are critical when preparing herbal remedies. Glass measuring cups and spoons are easy to clean and do not react with herbs or oils.

Labels and Markers

Proper labeling of herbal preparations is essential for safety and identification. Use waterproof labels and permanent markers to ensure the information stays intact.

Reference Books and Resources

A library of herbal reference books, websites, and reputable sources is indispensable for research, formulation, and ensuring the safe and effective use of herbs.

Safety Gear

When working with concentrated herbal extracts, safety gear like gloves and safety goggles is essential to protect against skin contact or splashes.

Herb Garden or Reliable Suppliers

For those who wish to grow their own herbs, an herb garden is a valuable resource. If not, establishing relationships with reliable herb suppliers is crucial to ensure the quality and authenticity of the herbs you use.

Herbal Identification Guides

To avoid misidentification and ensure you're using the correct plants, invest in reliable herbal identification guides or take courses on plant identification.

Straining Equipment

Depending on the preparation, you may need various straining tools, such as fine mesh sieves, nut milk bags, or specialized herbal strainers.

Glass Droppers and Pipettes

These tools are essential for precise measurements and dosing when working with liquid herbal extracts and tinctures.

Herb Scissors or Shears

Herb scissors or shears with multiple blades are handy for quickly chopping fresh herbs for teas, culinary use, or tincture preparation.

Storage Space

Having a designated and organized storage space for your dried herbs, tinctures, salves, and other herbal creations helps maintain their quality and accessibility.

Herb Press

A herb press is used to extract the maximum amount of liquid from herbal infusions or decoctions. It ensures that you get the most out of your herbs, especially when making herbal remedies in large quantities.

Dehydrator

While air drying is a traditional method for drying herbs, a dehydrator can expedite the process and help maintain the herbs' quality. It's particularly useful if you're working with a high volume of herbs or live in a humid climate.

Herb Grinder and Sifter

For making herbal capsules or powdered herbal preparations, an herb grinder and sifter combo is an efficient tool. It grinds herbs to a fine consistency and sifts out any larger particles, ensuring uniformity.

Herb Press

A herb press, also known as a tincture press, is used to extract the maximum amount of liquid from herbs when making tinctures or extracting herbal essences. It helps yield a more potent and concentrated final product.

pH Test Strips

pH test strips are essential for monitoring the pH levels of herbal preparations, especially when making creams, lotions, or other topical products. Correct pH is crucial to maintain the stability and effectiveness of these preparations.

Herbal Formulation Software

For advanced herbalists and practitioners, herbal formulation software can be a valuable tool. It assists in creating precise formulations and calculating herb proportions for specific remedies.

Herbal Containers and Packaging Materials

Consider the appropriate containers and packaging materials for your herbal products, whether you're selling them or giving them as gifts. This includes glass bottles for tinctures, jars for salves, and labels to provide information and branding.

Herbal Preparation Workstations

Having a dedicated space or workstation for herbal preparation ensures cleanliness and organization. It's important to separate your herbal preparation area from other activities to prevent cross-contamination.

Pest Control Measures

If you're growing your herbs, pest control measures such as organic pesticides or companion planting can help protect your plants from pests and maintain their health.

Water Filtration System

If you're using tap water in your herbal preparations, a water filtration system can help remove impurities and chemicals, ensuring the purity of your remedies.

Herbal Labeling Software

For herbalists or businesses that produce herbal products on a larger scale, specialized herbal labeling software can streamline the process of creating professional labels for your products. This software often includes templates and regulatory compliance features to ensure accurate and informative labeling.

Herb Drying Shed or Space

If you're growing and drying herbs in larger quantities, a dedicated drying shed or ample drying space is beneficial. This allows you to efficiently dry herbs in controlled conditions, ensuring optimal preservation of their properties.

Herb Identification Apps

In the age of technology, herb identification apps can be valuable resources. These apps use image recognition and databases to help you identify plants in the wild or in your garden, reducing the risk of misidentification.

Herbal Education Courses

Investing in herbal education courses, workshops, or certifications can provide you with a deeper understanding of herbal medicine, plant identification, ethical harvesting practices, and formulation techniques. Continuous learning is essential for mastering the art of herbalism.

Herbal Consultation Space

If you plan to offer herbal consultations or run a practice, having a dedicated and comfortable consultation space is essential for meeting with clients, discussing health concerns, and providing personalized herbal recommendations.

Herb Press and Infusion Bags

A herb press, combined with infusion bags, can simplify the process of extracting liquid from herbal infusions. It ensures maximum yield and potency when making large batches of herbal extracts or tinctures.

Herb Sourcing Knowledge

Developing knowledge about where and how to source high-quality herbs is crucial. Understanding the difference between wildcrafted, organic, and conventionally grown herbs, as well as reputable suppliers, ensures that you use the best-quality ingredients in your herbal preparations.

Herbal Hydrosols

Herbal hydrosols are byproducts of the steam distillation process used to make essential oils. They are gentle, aromatic waters with subtle herbal properties and can be used in skincare products, aromatic sprays, or as ingredients in herbal recipes.

Herbal Incense and Smudging Materials

Incense and smudging materials, such as sage bundles or palo santo sticks, can be used for cleansing spaces, promoting relaxation, and adding a spiritual or ceremonial aspect to herbal practices.

Chapter 12: Techniques of Extraction and Preparation

In the world of herbal medicine, mastering various techniques of extraction and preparation is essential for creating effective and safe herbal remedies. This chapter explores the key methods used to extract the therapeutic properties of herbs and how to prepare them for various applications.

Infusions

Infusions involve steeping herbs in hot water to extract their medicinal compounds. There are two primary types of infusions:

Herbal Tea: The most common form of infusion, herbal teas are prepared by pouring hot water over dried or fresh herbs. Cover and let steep for the desired time, typically 10-15 minutes.

Decoctions: Decoctions are used for tougher plant materials like roots and bark. Boil the herbs in water for a longer time, typically 15-20 minutes, to extract their active constituents fully.

Tinctures

Tinctures are concentrated herbal extracts created by steeping herbs in alcohol or glycerin. To prepare a tincture:

- Finely chop or grind the dried herb.
- Place the herb in a glass jar.
- Cover with alcohol (typically vodka or brandy) or glycerin.
- Seal the jar and let it sit for several weeks, shaking it regularly.
- Strain the liquid, and the resulting tincture is ready for use.

Infused Oils

Infused oils are made by extracting the medicinal properties of herbs into a carrier oil, such as olive or almond oil. To make an infused oil:

- Fill a glass jar with dried herbs.
- Cover the herbs with the chosen carrier oil.
- Seal the jar and place it in a sunny spot for 2-6 weeks, shaking it occasionally.
- Strain the oil, and it's ready for use in salves, massage oils, or as a base for various herbal products.

Salves

Salves are semi-solid herbal preparations used for topical applications. To make a salve:

- Create an herbal-infused oil as described above.
- Melt beeswax in a double boiler.
- Add the herbal-infused oil to the melted beeswax.
- Stir until well combined, and pour the mixture into containers to solidify.

Poultices

Poultices are herbal preparations used for localized applications. To make a poultice:

- Blend or crush fresh or dried herbs.
- Add enough warm water or other liquid to create a thick, moist paste.
- Apply the paste directly to the affected area.
- Cover with a clean cloth or bandage.

Capsules

Capsules are a convenient way to take powdered herbs, especially if the taste is unpalatable. You can purchase empty gelatin or vegetarian capsules and fill them with powdered herbs using a capsule-filling machine.

Syrups

Syrups are sweet, herbal preparations often used for respiratory or immune support. To make an herbal syrup:

- Create a strong herbal infusion or decoction.
- Strain the liquid and return it to the heat.
- Add honey or another sweetener and simmer until it thickens.
- Pour into bottles and store in the refrigerator.

Herbal Baths

Herbal baths involve steeping herbs in hot water and adding the infusion to bathwater for relaxation and skin benefits. Place herbs in a cloth bag or directly in the bathwater.

Steam Inhalations

Steam inhalations are useful for respiratory conditions. To prepare a steam inhalation:

- Boil water and pour it into a bowl.
- Add dried herbs like eucalyptus or chamomile.
- Lean over the bowl with a towel over your head to inhale the steam.

Herbal Compresses

Herbal compresses involve applying a cloth soaked in a strong herbal infusion or decoction to the affected area. This method is often used for external pain relief, muscle relaxation, or wound care.

- Prepare a strong herbal infusion or decoction.
- Soak a clean cloth in the herbal liquid.
- Apply the soaked cloth to the skin, covering the area of concern.
- Leave the compress in place for the desired duration.

Herbal Elixirs

Herbal elixirs are sweet or syrupy preparations that combine herbal infusions or tinctures with honey, glycerin, or other sweeteners. They are a convenient way to administer herbs to children or those who dislike the taste of tinctures.

- Prepare an herbal infusion or tincture.
- Mix it with a sweetener of choice, such as honey or glycerin.
- Store the elixir in a glass bottle and label it for easy identification.

Herbal Steams

Herbal steams are used for facial treatments or respiratory relief. To prepare an herbal steam:

- Boil water and pour it into a bowl.
- Add dried herbs like lavender, chamomile, or eucalyptus.
- Cover your head with a towel and lean over the bowl to inhale the steam.

Herbal Mouthwashes and Gargles

Herbal mouthwashes and gargles are beneficial for oral hygiene and throat discomfort. To make an herbal mouthwash or gargle:

- Create a strong herbal infusion or decoction, often using herbs like sage, thyme, or calendula.
- Allow it to cool to room temperature.
- Gargle or rinse your mouth with the herbal liquid.

Herbal Foot Soaks

Herbal foot soaks are relaxing and can be used to address foot-related issues like athlete's foot or general fatigue. To prepare a foot soak:

- Create a strong herbal infusion or decoction.
- Pour it into a basin or foot bath filled with warm water.
- Soak your feet in the herbal mixture for a specified time.

Herbal Smoke

While not as common, some traditional practices involve **herbal smoke** for ritual or medicinal purposes. Herbs like white sage or cedar are dried and burned to release aromatic smoke.

Herbal Suppositories

Herbal suppositories are used for rectal or vaginal applications. They involve combining herbal-infused oils with a solidifying agent like cocoa butter, which is then shaped into suppositories for insertion.

Herbal Sitz Baths

Sitz baths are used for soothing conditions related to the pelvic area, such as hemorrhoids or postpartum discomfort. Herbal infusions or decoctions are added to warm water in a special basin or tub for soaking.

Herbal Liniments

Herbal liniments are liquid topical preparations used for muscle pain or external injuries. They are typically alcohol-based and may contain herbs like arnica or comfrey.

Herbal Mouth Sprays

Herbal mouth sprays can offer quick relief for sore throats or oral discomfort. They are made by combining herbal tinctures with water or glycerin and then spraying them directly into the mouth.

Herbal Capsules and Tablets

Herbal capsules and tablets provide a convenient and precise way to take herbal remedies, especially if the taste or texture of certain herbs is unpalatable. These are made by encapsulating powdered herbs in gelatin or vegetarian capsules or compressing them into tablets.

- Powder the dried herbs finely.
- Fill empty capsules or tablet press molds with the powdered herbs.
- Seal the capsules or allow the tablets to dry and harden.
- Label and store in a cool, dry place.

Herbal Sprays

Herbal sprays are used for various purposes, such as soothing skin irritations, freshening the air, or providing aromatherapy benefits. These are made by combining herbal infusions, tinctures, or essential oils with distilled water.

- Prepare the herbal infusion, tincture, or essential oil blend.
- Dilute it with distilled water to the desired concentration.
- Transfer the mixture into a spray bottle.
- Label the bottle for easy identification.

Herbal Bath Bombs

Herbal bath bombs are effervescent bath products that release herbs and essential oils into the bathwater for relaxation and therapeutic benefits. They can be made by combining baking soda, citric acid, and herbs infused in carrier oil.

- Mix baking soda and citric acid in a bowl.
- Add herbal-infused oil and any desired essential oils.
- Shape the mixture into bath bomb molds and allow them to dry.
- Store in an airtight container.

Herbal Honey

Herbal honey is a delicious way to enjoy the benefits of herbs and can be used in teas, on toast, or in recipes. It's made by infusing dried herbs in honey.

- Fill a glass jar with dried herbs.
- Pour honey over the herbs, ensuring they are fully covered.
- Seal the jar and let it sit for several weeks, stirring occasionally.
- Strain the honey, removing the herbs, and store it in a clean jar.

Herbal Ferments

Fermentation is used to create herbal ferments like herbal kefir, kombucha, or fermented herbal drinks. These can provide probiotic and digestive benefits.

- Prepare an herbal infusion or decoction.
- Allow it to cool to room temperature.
- Add a starter culture like kefir grains or kombucha SCOBY.
- Allow the mixture to ferment for the specified time, usually several days to weeks.

Herbal Vinegars

Herbal vinegars are made by infusing herbs in vinegar, which can be used in salad dressings, culinary recipes, or as a digestive tonic.

- Fill a glass jar with dried or fresh herbs.
- Cover the herbs with vinegar (typically apple cider vinegar).
- Seal the jar and let it sit in a dark place for several weeks.
- Strain the vinegar, and it's ready for use.

Herbal Honeys and Syrups for Cough and Cold

Herbal honeys and syrups are made by infusing herbs known for their cough and cold-relieving properties into honey or sugar syrup. These can provide relief from respiratory symptoms.

- sCreate a strong herbal infusion or decoction.
- Strain the liquid.
- Mix the herbal liquid with honey or sugar syrup.
- Store in a glass container and label it for use during coughs and colds.

Chapter 13: Making Herbal Salves, Balms, and Ointments

Herbal salves, balms, and ointments are topical preparations that offer a soothing and healing application for various skin conditions, wounds, and muscle discomfort. This chapter delves into the art of crafting these herbal remedies, providing insights into the ingredients and techniques involved.

Ingredients for Herbal Salves, Balms, and Ointments

Herbs: Select dried or fresh herbs that have specific properties for your intended purpose. Calendula, comfrey, lavender, and plantain are popular choices.

Carrier Oil: Choose a carrier oil like olive oil, coconut oil, or sweet almond oil. The carrier oil acts as the base and extracts the medicinal properties of the herbs.

Beeswax: Beeswax is used to thicken and solidify the salve, balm, or ointment. It also helps create a protective barrier on the skin.

Essential Oils: Essential oils can enhance the healing properties and aroma of your preparation. For example, lavender essential oil is soothing, while tea tree oil has antibacterial properties.

Vitamin E Oil: Vitamin E oil is often added as a natural preservative and skin-nourishing ingredient.

Steps to Make Herbal Salves, Balms, and Ointments

Infusing Herbs: Begin by infusing the herbs into the carrier oil. This process allows the oil to absorb the therapeutic compounds from the herbs.

Place the chosen herbs in a clean, dry glass jar.

Cover the herbs completely with the carrier oil.

Seal the jar tightly and place it in a warm, sunny location for several weeks. Alternatively, you can use gentle heat, such as a double boiler, to speed up the infusion process.

Straining: After the infusion period, strain the oil to remove the herbal material. This leaves you with a potent herbal-infused oil as the base of your salve, balm, or ointment.

Melting Beeswax: In a double boiler, gently melt the beeswax. The amount of beeswax you use will determine the consistency of your final product. More beeswax results in a firmer salve, while less creates a softer balm.

Blending: Combine the herbal-infused oil with the melted beeswax. Stir well to ensure a uniform mixture.

Adding Essential Oils and Vitamin E: If desired, add a few drops of essential oils for fragrance and added therapeutic benefits. Also, mix in vitamin E oil as a natural preservative.

Pouring and Cooling: Carefully pour the hot mixture into clean, dry containers, such as small jars or tins. Allow it to cool and solidify.

Labeling: Label each container with the name of the salve, balm, or ointment, along with the date of preparation and a list of ingredients used.

Tips and Considerations

Experiment with different herbs and essential oils to create formulations tailored to specific skin concerns, such as soothing chamomile for sensitive skin or anti-inflammatory arnica for muscle relief.

Maintain cleanliness throughout the preparation process to prevent contamination of your herbal products.

Store your herbal salves, balms, and ointments in a cool, dark place to prolong their shelf life and efficacy.

Perform a patch test before applying any new herbal product to a larger area of skin to check for allergic reactions or sensitivities.

Be aware of the shelf life of your herbal creations, as they may vary depending on the ingredients used. Vitamin E oil can help extend the product's freshness.

Troubleshooting and Customization:

Adjusting Consistency: The amount of beeswax you use will determine the texture of your salve. If it's too soft, add more melted beeswax; if it's too firm, add more herbal-infused oil.

Customizing Scents: The choice of essential oils not only affects the aroma but also adds therapeutic benefits. Lavender essential oil promotes relaxation, while tea tree oil has antimicrobial properties. Experiment with different combinations to create the desired scent profile and therapeutic effects.

Adding Additional Ingredients: Depending on the intended use of your salve, you can incorporate other beneficial ingredients such as shea butter for extra moisturization or aloe vera gel for soothing properties.

Application and Usage:

Cleanse the Skin: Before applying the herbal salve, ensure that the skin is clean and dry. Gently wash the affected area and pat it dry with a clean towel.

Apply Sparingly: A little goes a long way with herbal salves. Use a small amount and gently massage it into the skin until absorbed. For ointments or balms, apply a thin layer.

Frequency: Follow the recommended application frequency for your specific herbal preparation. Some may be applied several times a day, while others are best used as needed.

Storage: Store your herbal salves, balms, and ointments in a cool, dark place to maintain their potency. Avoid exposing them to excessive heat or sunlight.

Labeling and Safety:

Label Clearly: Ensure that each container is labeled clearly with the name of the product, the date of preparation, and a list of ingredients. This is important for easy identification and safety.

Allergy and Sensitivity: Be mindful of potential allergies or sensitivities to the herbs or essential oils used in your preparation. Perform a patch test on a small area of skin before widespread use.

Sharing Your Herbal Creations:

Gifts and Personal Use: Herbal salves, balms, and ointments make thoughtful gifts for friends and family. They can also become essential components of your personal wellness toolkit.

Selling Your Products: If you plan to sell your herbal creations, research local regulations and consider liability insurance. Ensure that your labeling and product descriptions comply with legal requirements.

Educating Yourself Continuously:

Stay Informed: Herbalism is a continually evolving field. Stay updated on the latest research, safety guidelines, and best practices for working with herbs.

Herbal Courses: Consider taking herbal courses or workshops to deepen your knowledge and gain practical skills in herbal preparation.

Safety Considerations:

Avoid Contamination: When making herbal salves, cleanliness is crucial. Use sterilized equipment and containers to prevent contamination. Even a small amount of moisture or foreign matter can spoil your preparation.

Allergies and Sensitivities: Be aware of potential allergies or sensitivities to herbs, carrier oils, beeswax, or essential oils. Perform patch tests on a small area of skin before applying the product more widely, especially if you plan to share it with others.

Storage and Shelf Life: Properly store your herbal salves, balms, and ointments in airtight containers in a cool, dark place. This helps maintain their shelf life, which can vary depending on the ingredients used. Adding vitamin E oil as a natural preservative can extend their freshness.

Labeling and Documentation:

Accurate Labeling: Ensure that each container is labeled accurately and comprehensively. Include the name of the product, date of preparation, and a detailed list of ingredients. This is not only essential for easy identification but also for safety and regulatory compliance if you plan to sell your creations.

Documentation: Keep records of your recipes and formulations. This documentation can be valuable for replicating successful products and troubleshooting any issues that may arise.

Exploring Advanced Formulations:

Specialized Salves: As you gain expertise, you can explore specialized herbal salves for specific purposes. For example, you might create a salve for joint pain with herbs like arnica and ginger or a soothing salve for insect bites and stings with herbs like plantain and chamomile.

Customized Blends: Consider blending multiple herbal-infused oils and essential oils to create unique formulations that address a combination of skin or health concerns.

Sharing Your Knowledge:

Teaching Workshops: If you become proficient in herbal preparation, you can consider teaching workshops or classes to share your knowledge and passion for herbalism with others.

Community Engagement: Engage with your local community or online herbalist communities to exchange ideas, experiences, and insights with fellow herbalists and enthusiasts.

Ethical and Sustainable Practices:

Sourcing Herbs: When sourcing herbs, consider ethical and sustainable practices. Support local growers or harvest wild plants responsibly, ensuring that you're not depleting natural resources.

Respect for Nature: Foster a deep respect for nature and the plants you work with. Cultivate an eco-conscious mindset in your herbal practice, minimizing waste and using resources wisely.

Chapter 14: Crafting Herbal Pills, Capsules, and Powders

Herbal pills, capsules, and powders offer a convenient and precise way to administer herbs, especially for those who prefer not to consume herbal teas or tinctures. In this chapter, we'll explore the art of crafting these herbal preparations, including the ingredients, methods, and considerations involved.

Ingredients for Herbal Pills, Capsules, and Powders

Dried Herbs: Choose high-quality dried herbs that are suitable for your intended purpose. The choice of herbs depends on the desired therapeutic effects.

Capsules or Gelatin Capsules: You can purchase empty gelatin or vegetarian capsules in various sizes. Capsules are ideal for encapsulating powdered herbs.

Steps to Craft Herbal Pills, Capsules, and Powders

1. Herb Preparation:

Powdering Herbs: To create herbal powders, you'll need to grind dried herbs into a fine powder. You can use a mortar and pestle or an electric herb grinder for this purpose.

Sourcing Pre-Powdered Herbs: Alternatively, you can source pre-powdered herbs if you prefer not to do the grinding yourself.

2. Filling Capsules:

Select the Appropriate Capsule Size: Choose the capsule size that suits your needs. Typically, size "0" or "00" capsules are used for encapsulating powdered herbs.

Fill the Capsules: Open each capsule and fill it with the powdered herb using a capsule-filling machine or by hand. Ensure that the capsules are evenly filled but not overstuffed.

Seal the Capsules: Reassemble the filled capsules by pressing the halves together until they snap into place.

3. Labeling and Storage:

Label Clearly: Label the containers of your herbal pills, capsules, or powders with the name of the product, the date of preparation, and a list of ingredients. This is important for easy identification and safety.

Storage: Store your herbal preparations in a cool, dry place to maintain their potency. Use airtight containers to prevent exposure to moisture and light.

Considerations for Crafting Herbal Pills, Capsules, and Powders

Dosage Accuracy: When crafting herbal pills, capsules, or powders, it's essential to accurately measure the dosage for each unit. This ensures that users receive a consistent and effective amount of the herb.

Individualized Formulas: Depending on your expertise and objectives, you can create customized herbal formulas by blending multiple powdered herbs in specific proportions. This allows you to tailor your preparations to address unique health concerns.

Quality Control: Source herbs from reputable suppliers to ensure their quality and purity. Conduct quality control checks to verify that the herbs meet your standards before using them in your preparations.

Allergen Awareness: Be aware of potential allergens in your herbal preparations, especially if you plan to share them with others. Clearly label any potential allergens, such as tree nuts or gluten, on your products.

Educational Resources: Continuously educate yourself about the properties and safety considerations of the herbs you work with. Stay informed about any potential contraindications or interactions with medications.

Precision and Consistency: One of the primary advantages of herbal pills, capsules, and powders is the ability to provide precise and consistent dosages. This is particularly important in herbal medicine, where the therapeutic effect often depends on the amount of the active compounds administered. Crafting these preparations allows for accurate dosing, ensuring that individuals receive the right amount of herbal remedy each time.

Taste and Convenience: Some individuals may find the taste of certain herbs unpleasant or challenging to tolerate in the form of teas or tinctures. Herbal pills, capsules, and powders offer an excellent alternative, as they allow people to bypass the taste while still benefiting from the herbs' therapeutic properties. This is especially helpful for herbs with bitter or strong flavors.

Portability: Herbal pills, capsules, and powders are highly portable, making them convenient for on-the-go use. Individuals can easily carry their herbal remedies in a purse, backpack, or travel bag, ensuring they have access to their chosen herbs wherever they are.

Longer Shelf Life: Properly prepared and stored herbal pills, capsules, and powders tend to have a longer shelf life compared to herbal tinctures or teas. This longevity makes them suitable for stocking up on herbs or creating herbal preparations that can be used over an extended period.

Custom Formulations: Crafting your herbal pills, capsules, and powders gives you the flexibility to create custom formulations tailored to individual health needs. You can blend specific herbs to address multiple aspects of a person's health or create unique herbal formulas for specific conditions.

Avoiding Additives: When you make your herbal pills and capsules, you have control over the ingredients. This means you can avoid common additives or fillers that may be present in commercially manufactured herbal supplements.

Educational Tool: Crafting herbal pills, capsules, and powders can serve as an educational tool. You can teach others about the benefits of herbal medicine, demonstrate the preparation process, and empower them to take an active role in their health and wellness.

Quality Assurance: By preparing herbal remedies yourself, you can ensure the quality and purity of the herbs used. This is especially important if you have concerns about the sourcing and processing of commercially available herbal products.

Respecting Tradition: The art of crafting herbal pills, capsules, and powders connects you with a rich tradition of herbalism that spans cultures and centuries. It allows you to embrace and continue this ancient practice in a modern context.

Regulatory Considerations: When crafting herbal pills, capsules, and powders for sale or distribution, it's essential to be aware of the regulatory requirements in your region or country. Different jurisdictions may have specific rules and standards governing the production, labeling, and marketing of herbal supplements. Ensure that your products comply with these regulations to maintain legality and consumer safety.

Testing and Quality Control: Implement quality control measures to verify the identity, purity, and potency of the herbs you use. Consider working with a reputable laboratory to conduct testing, including organoleptic evaluation, microscopic analysis, and chemical assays. This ensures that your herbal preparations meet the highest quality standards.

Ethical Sourcing and Sustainability: Be mindful of where and how you source your herbs. Supporting ethical and sustainable practices is not only responsible but also reflects positively on your herbal brand. Consider practices such as wildcrafting herbs responsibly, sourcing from organic growers, and promoting fair trade principles.

Label Transparency: Transparent and informative labeling is crucial for herbal pills, capsules, and powders. Provide clear and accurate information about the ingredients used, dosage instructions, potential allergens, and any contraindications or precautions. Labeling should also include contact information and, if applicable, regulatory compliance details.

Batch Records and Traceability: Maintain meticulous batch records for each production run of your herbal preparations. These records should include details about the herbs used, their sources, processing methods, and quality control checks. Effective batch tracking and traceability systems help you respond to any quality or safety issues swiftly.

Educational Resources: If you intend to distribute or sell your herbal products, consider providing educational resources to your customers. Information about the herbs' properties, usage, and potential benefits can empower individuals to make informed choices and use the products effectively.

Packaging and Presentation: The packaging and presentation of your herbal pills, capsules, and powders play a role in the overall appeal of your products. Choose packaging that preserves the integrity of the herbs and protects them from moisture and light. Thoughtful presentation enhances the perceived value of your herbal preparations.

Collaboration and Networking: Building connections within the herbal community can be valuable for sharing knowledge, sourcing herbs, and gaining insights into best practices. Consider joining herbalist associations, attending conferences, or participating in online forums to network with fellow herbalists and enthusiasts.

Continuous Learning: Herbalism is a lifelong journey of learning and discovery. Stay updated on the latest research, herbal trends, and advancements in the field. This ongoing education ensures that your herbal preparations remain relevant and effective.

Ethical Marketing: When promoting your herbal products, practice ethical marketing. Avoid making exaggerated claims or promising unrealistic results. Instead, focus on providing accurate information and fostering trust with your customers.

Chapter 15: Storage and Shelf Life: Keeping Remedies Potent

Effective storage is crucial in maintaining the potency and safety of herbal remedies. In this chapter, we will explore the factors that influence the shelf life of herbal preparations, how to store them correctly, and strategies to extend their freshness.

Factors Affecting Shelf Life of Herbal Preparations

Ingredient Quality: The quality of the herbs and ingredients used in your herbal remedies significantly impacts their shelf life. Fresh, high-quality herbs tend to maintain their potency longer than herbs that have been poorly harvested or stored.

Exposure to Light: Light exposure can cause herbs to deteriorate and lose their efficacy. Store herbal remedies in opaque containers or in a cool, dark place to minimize light exposure.

Moisture and Humidity: Moisture can lead to mold, spoilage, and degradation of herbal remedies. Keep herbal preparations in airtight containers to prevent moisture from entering.

Temperature: Temperature fluctuations can cause herbs to deteriorate rapidly. Store herbal remedies in a cool, consistent temperature environment to prolong their shelf life. Avoid exposing them to extreme heat or cold.

Oxygen Exposure: Oxygen can lead to oxidation, which may degrade the active compounds in herbs. Use airtight containers to minimize oxygen exposure and consider adding oxygen-absorbing packets to long-term storage containers.

Contamination: Properly sterilize containers and equipment to prevent contamination. Ensure that your hands are clean when handling herbal preparations to avoid introducing bacteria or pathogens.

Storage Guidelines for Herbal Remedies

Use Airtight Containers: Store herbal remedies in airtight containers to prevent exposure to oxygen and moisture. Glass containers with tight-sealing lids are often a good choice.

Keep It Cool: Store herbal preparations in a cool, dark place. A consistent temperature between 50°F to 70°F (10°C to 21°C) is ideal. Avoid storing them in direct sunlight, near heat sources, or in humid environments like the bathroom.

Label Clearly: Label each container with the name of the product, the date of preparation, and a list of ingredients. Clear labeling helps you keep track of the age of your remedies and ensures proper usage.

Monitor for Signs of Spoilage: Regularly check herbal preparations for any signs of spoilage, such as mold, off odors, or changes in color or texture. Discard any remedies that show these signs.

Use Oxygen Absorbers: In long-term storage, consider using oxygen-absorbing packets to remove excess oxygen from containers. This can help extend the shelf life of your remedies.

Rotate Stock: If you have a large herbal inventory, use the "first in, first out" (FIFO) method to ensure that older remedies are used before newer ones. This helps prevent remedies from sitting unused for extended periods.

Extending Shelf Life Through Preservation Methods

Drying Herbs: Drying herbs thoroughly before using them in preparations can significantly extend their shelf life. This applies to both dried herbs and fresh herbs you intend to use for infusions or tinctures.

Alcohol-Based Tinctures: Alcohol-based tinctures have a longer shelf life compared to water-based ones. The alcohol acts as a preservative, preventing the growth of microorganisms.

Adding Natural Preservatives: Some herbal preparations benefit from the addition of natural preservatives like vitamin E oil or grapefruit seed extract. These can help extend shelf life.

Refrigeration or Freezing: In some cases, refrigeration or freezing may be suitable for specific herbal preparations, such as herbal oils or salves, to prevent rancidity or spoilage.

Transparency and Labelling: Clearly label your herbal remedies with essential information such as the product name, date of preparation, and a detailed list of ingredients. This labeling not only helps you keep track of your preparations but also informs users about what they are using. It's a critical safety measure, especially if you share or sell your remedies.

Storage Containers: The choice of storage containers is crucial. Glass containers with tight-sealing lids are often recommended because they are less permeable than plastic, which can prevent the escape of volatile aromatic compounds and maintain the freshness of your remedies. Ensure the containers are clean and dry before filling them.

Protection from Light: Light can degrade the active compounds in herbs and herbal preparations. Therefore, it's essential to store your remedies in opaque containers or dark-colored glass bottles to protect them from light exposure. Avoid clear or translucent containers unless they are stored in a dark place.

Moisture Control: Moisture is a common enemy of herbal remedies as it can lead to mold growth, spoilage, and loss of efficacy. Always store your herbal preparations in a dry environment. If moisture is a concern, consider adding a desiccant or moisture-absorbing packet to the container.

Herbal Oil Infusions: If you are working with herbal oils or infused oils, keep them in the refrigerator to prevent rancidity. Oils are sensitive to temperature fluctuations, and refrigeration helps maintain their freshness.

Check for Signs of Spoilage: Periodically inspect your herbal remedies for any signs of spoilage or degradation. Look for mold growth, unusual odors, changes in color or texture, or the presence of visible contaminants. If any of these signs are present, discard the preparation.

Long-Term Storage: If you plan to store herbal remedies for an extended period, consider vacuum sealing or using canning jars with vacuum-sealed lids to remove oxygen from the container. This can significantly extend the shelf life of your remedies.

Regular Inventory Rotation: To ensure you use your herbal preparations before they expire, practice regular inventory rotation. Use the "first in, first out" (FIFO) method, where you use the oldest remedies first. This reduces the risk of remedies sitting unused for extended periods.

Documentation: Maintain detailed records of your herbal preparations, including the recipes used, the sources of your herbs, the preparation dates, and any quality control measures you employed. This documentation can be invaluable for troubleshooting and quality assurance.

Environmental Considerations: In addition to preserving the shelf life of your remedies, consider environmentally friendly practices. Opt for sustainable packaging, minimize waste, and support ethical sourcing of herbs to reduce your impact on the environment.

Sharing Knowledge: Educate those who use your remedies about proper storage and shelf life. Providing guidelines and information on how to store and handle herbal preparations ensures that individuals can benefit from them effectively and safely.

4. Essential Oils 101: Extraction, Benefits, and Uses

Chapter 16: Distillation: The Science Behind Essential Oils

Distillation is a fundamental process in the production of essential oils, which are highly concentrated extracts of aromatic compounds from plants. In this chapter, we'll explore the science behind distillation, the equipment involved, and the principles that make it possible to capture the essence of plants in the form of essential oils.

The Essence of Distillation

At its core, distillation is a separation process that takes advantage of differences in boiling points to isolate and capture specific substances from a mixture. In the context of essential oil production, distillation is used to separate the volatile aromatic compounds from plant material, resulting in highly concentrated essential oils.

The Distillation Process

The distillation process for essential oils typically involves the following steps:

Plant Material Preparation: High-quality plant material is harvested, cleaned, and sometimes crushed or chopped to facilitate the release of aromatic compounds.

Loading the Still: The prepared plant material is loaded into a distillation apparatus called a still. There are different types of stills, including alembic stills, steam distillation units, and hydrodistillation units.

Heating: The still is heated, and the plant material undergoes a temperature-controlled process. The aromatic compounds within the plant material vaporize as they reach their respective boiling points.

Vaporization and Condensation: The vaporized aromatic compounds rise through the still, entering a cooling system or condenser, which cools the vapor and condenses it back into a liquid form.

Collection: The condensed liquid, now a mixture of water and essential oil, is collected in a separate container. Since essential oils are less dense than water, they float on top and can be easily separated.

Separation: The collected mixture is allowed to sit, and over time, the essential oil separates from the water phase. The oil is then carefully siphoned or drained off.

Key Factors in Distillation

Several factors influence the success of distillation for essential oil production:

Plant Selection: The choice of plant material is crucial. Different plants yield different amounts and qualities of essential oils. The timing of harvest can also impact oil quality.

Temperature Control: Precise temperature control is essential during distillation. High temperatures can cause thermal degradation of the aromatic compounds, while low temperatures may not effectively release them.

Duration: The duration of distillation varies depending on the plant material and the desired oil. Longer distillation times can sometimes yield more oil, but excessive duration can also degrade the oil's quality.

Quality of Equipment: The quality and design of the distillation apparatus, such as the type of still used, can impact the efficiency and quality of the process.

Water Quality: The quality of the water used in distillation can affect the final product. Pure, distilled water is typically used to avoid contamination of the essential oil.

Applications of Essential Oils

Essential oils extracted through distillation have a wide range of applications, including aromatherapy, perfumery, natural cosmetics, and therapeutic uses. Each essential oil has its unique aroma and potential health benefits based on the specific aromatic compounds it contains.

Variations in Distillation Techniques: While the basic principles of distillation remain the same, there are variations in techniques depending on the plant material and desired outcome:

Steam Distillation: This is one of the most common methods for extracting essential oils. Steam is passed through the plant material, vaporizing the aromatic compounds, and then condensing them.

Hydrodistillation: Similar to steam distillation but uses water as the solvent instead of steam. It is often used for tougher plant materials.

Fractional Distillation: This technique is employed to separate different constituents of essential oils based on their boiling points. It allows for the isolation of specific compounds.

Fractional Distillation: This technique is employed to separate different constituents of essential oils based on their boiling points. It allows for the isolation of specific compounds.

Quality Control: Ensuring the quality of essential oils is crucial. Factors such as the time of harvest, the part of the plant used, and the distillation process itself can impact the final product. Proper quality control measures, including testing for purity and authenticity, help maintain the integrity of essential oils.

Sustainability: The growing demand for essential oils has raised concerns about sustainability. Ethical practices, such as sustainable sourcing, responsible harvesting, and supporting fair trade initiatives, are essential to ensure that essential oil production does not harm ecosystems or local communities.

Chemical Complexity: Essential oils are complex mixtures of volatile compounds, including terpenes, phenols, aldehydes, and esters. These compounds contribute to the aroma and therapeutic properties of the oil. Understanding the chemical composition of essential oils is crucial for their safe and effective use.

Aromatherapy: Essential oils are widely used in aromatherapy, where the inhalation or topical application of these oils is believed to have therapeutic effects on physical, emotional, and mental well-being. Each essential oil has its unique scent and potential therapeutic properties, making aromatherapy a holistic practice.

Traditional and Modern Medicine: Essential oils have been used in traditional medicine systems for centuries. Today, they find applications in modern medicine, including in the development of pharmaceuticals and as complementary therapies.

Research and Innovation: Ongoing research in the field of essential oils continues to uncover new potential benefits and applications. Scientists are exploring their antimicrobial, anti-inflammatory, and antioxidant properties, among others.

Safety Considerations: Essential oils are potent and should be used with caution. They can cause skin irritation, allergic reactions, or adverse effects if not used properly. Dilution and adherence to recommended usage guidelines are essential for safety.

Chapter 17: Therapeutic Benefits of Top Essential Oils

Essential oils, derived through distillation, are celebrated for their therapeutic properties in various wellness practices, including aromatherapy, holistic medicine, and skincare. In this chapter, we will explore the therapeutic benefits of some of the most commonly used essential oils.

Lavender Essential Oil

Lavender oil is one of the most versatile and popular essential oils, known for its calming and soothing effects. Its therapeutic benefits include:

Relaxation: Lavender oil is renowned for its ability to reduce stress and anxiety. Inhaling its aroma or adding it to a diffuser can promote relaxation and improve sleep quality.

Skin Health: Lavender oil has antiseptic and anti-inflammatory properties, making it beneficial for treating minor burns, cuts, and insect bites. It's also used in skincare products to soothe and hydrate the skin.

Pain Relief: When applied topically, lavender oil may provide relief from headaches, muscle aches, and joint pain.

Peppermint Essential Oil

Peppermint oil has a refreshing and invigorating scent and offers several therapeutic benefits:

Digestive Aid: Peppermint oil can help alleviate indigestion, bloating, and nausea when diluted and applied topically or inhaled. It can also be added to teas for digestive support.

Headache Relief: Applying diluted peppermint oil to the temples and forehead may reduce tension headaches and migraines.

Energy Booster: Inhaling the aroma of peppermint oil can increase alertness and energy levels, making it a great choice for a quick pick-me-up.

Tea Tree Essential Oil

Tea tree oil, with its distinct medicinal aroma, is known for its antibacterial and antifungal properties:

Skin Health: Tea tree oil is commonly used to treat acne, skin infections, and fungal conditions like athlete's foot and nail fungus. It can be applied topically, but always dilute it with a carrier oil.

Respiratory Health: Inhalation of tea tree oil vapor may help relieve symptoms of respiratory conditions like congestion and coughs.

Household Cleaner: Tea tree oil is a natural disinfectant and can be used to make homemade cleaning solutions to kill germs and bacteria.

Eucalyptus Essential Oil

Eucalyptus oil has a fresh, invigorating scent and is known for its respiratory benefits:

Respiratory Health: Eucalyptus oil can help relieve symptoms of colds, coughs, and sinus congestion when inhaled or added to steam inhalation.

Immune Support: Due to its antimicrobial properties, eucalyptus oil is used in many over-the-counter cold and flu remedies.

Lemon Essential Oil

Lemon oil has a bright, uplifting scent and offers various therapeutic advantages:

Mood Enhancement: Lemon oil is known to uplift and improve mood. Diffusing its aroma can help reduce stress and boost mental clarity.

Antimicrobial: Lemon oil has natural antibacterial and antiviral properties. It can be used as a natural disinfectant in cleaning products.

Digestive Aid: Ingesting a small amount of food-grade lemon oil with water may support digestion and detoxification.

Chamomile Essential Oil

Chamomile oil, derived from both Roman and German chamomile plants, is valued for its calming and anti-inflammatory properties:

Sleep Aid: Chamomile oil is renowned for its ability to promote relaxation and improve sleep quality. It can be used in aromatherapy or added to a warm bath.

Skin Care: Chamomile oil is gentle and soothing for the skin. It can help reduce skin irritation, redness, and inflammation.

Rosemary Essential Oil

Rosemary oil is known for its invigorating and stimulating properties:

Cognitive Enhancement: Rosemary oil may improve cognitive function, memory, and concentration. Inhaling its aroma or using it in a diffuser can enhance mental clarity.

Hair and Scalp Health: Rosemary oil is used in hair care products for its potential to promote hair growth and improve scalp health. It can also help with dandruff and dryness.

Antioxidant: The oil contains antioxidants that can help protect cells from oxidative damage.

Chamomile Essential Oil

Chamomile oil, derived from both Roman and German chamomile plants, is valued for its calming and anti-inflammatory properties:

Gentle for Sensitive Skin: Chamomile oil is suitable for sensitive skin and can help alleviate skin conditions like eczema and psoriasis.

Anti-Inflammatory: It can reduce skin inflammation and irritation, making it a popular choice in skincare products.

Digestive Health: Chamomile tea, made from chamomile flowers, is known to soothe digestive discomfort and promote relaxation.

Frankincense Essential Oil

Frankincense oil has been used for centuries for its potential health benefits:

Skin Rejuvenation: Frankincense oil is prized for its ability to rejuvenate the skin and reduce the appearance of wrinkles and scars.

Respiratory Support: Inhaling the aroma of frankincense oil may provide relief from respiratory issues like asthma and bronchitis.

Mood Elevation: It has a calming effect and is often used in meditation and relaxation practices to enhance spiritual and emotional well-being.

Geranium Essential Oil

Geranium oil is known for its floral and slightly sweet aroma:

Balancing Skin: Geranium oil is often used in skincare for its ability to balance oily and dry skin, reduce acne, and improve skin elasticity.

Mood Enhancement: It can help alleviate stress and anxiety and promote emotional stability when used in aromatherapy.

Insect Repellent: Geranium oil may act as a natural insect repellent when applied to the skin or diffused.

Ylang-Ylang Essential Oil

Ylang-ylang oil has a sweet and exotic fragrance:

Mood Upliftment: Ylang-ylang oil is known for its potential to reduce stress, improve mood, and promote relaxation. It is often used in perfumes and bath products.

Aphrodisiac: It is sometimes considered an aphrodisiac and is used to enhance sensuality and intimacy.

Hair Care: Ylang-ylang oil can be used in hair care products to promote healthy, shiny hair and a balanced scalp.

Safety Considerations

While essential oils offer numerous therapeutic benefits, it's essential to use them safely:

Dilution: Most essential oils should be diluted with a carrier oil (such as jojoba, coconut, or almond oil) before applying them to the skin to prevent irritation or sensitization.

Patch Test: Perform a patch test on a small area of skin to check for any adverse reactions before applying essential oils more extensively.

Consultation: If you have specific health concerns or are pregnant or nursing, consult a qualified practitioner or healthcare professional before using essential oils.

Quality: Ensure you are using high-quality, pure essential oils from reputable sources to reap their full therapeutic benefits.

Chapter 18: Safe Use and Dilution: Getting the Most Out of Oils

Essential oils are powerful and concentrated extracts, and their safe use and proper dilution are crucial to maximize their benefits while minimizing the risk of adverse reactions. In this chapter, we will delve into the principles of safe essential oil use and effective dilution techniques.

Understanding Essential Oil Potency

Essential oils are highly concentrated and potent extracts obtained from plant materials. They contain the aromatic compounds, natural chemicals, and volatile constituents that give plants their characteristic scents and therapeutic properties. Due to their potency, essential oils should be handled with care to ensure safety and efficacy.

Importance of Dilution

Dilution is the process of mixing essential oils with a carrier oil or another base to reduce their concentration before applying them to the skin. Dilution serves several important purposes:

Skin Safety: Essential oils in their undiluted form can be irritating or sensitizing to the skin. Dilution helps prevent skin reactions, such as redness, itching, or burning.

Even Distribution: Dilution ensures that essential oils are evenly distributed and absorbed by the skin, allowing for effective and controlled application.

Cost-Effective: Dilution extends the use of essential oils, as they are expensive due to the large quantities of plant material required for extraction.

Carrier Oils Carrier oils are neutral, non-volatile oils that are used to dilute essential oils. Some commonly used carrier oils include:

Jojoba Oil: Known for its similarity to the skin's natural oils, making it suitable for various skin types.

Coconut Oil: Has natural antimicrobial properties and is nourishing for the skin and hair.

Sweet Almond Oil: A gentle and versatile carrier oil often used in skincare.

Grapeseed Oil: Lightweight and easily absorbed, making it ideal for massage and blending with essential oils.

Guidelines for Safe Dilution

The appropriate dilution ratio depends on factors such as the essential oil used, the purpose of application, and individual skin sensitivity. Here are some general guidelines:

For Adults: A common dilution ratio for adults is 2-3% essential oil in a carrier oil. This equates to 2-3 drops of essential oil per teaspoon (5 mL) of carrier oil.

For Children and Sensitive Skin: When using essential oils on children, the elderly, or those with sensitive skin, it's advisable to use a lower dilution ratio, typically 1% or less.

Face and Sensitive Areas: Use a lower dilution ratio of around 1% for sensitive areas like the face, neck, and mucous membranes.

Specific Uses: Some applications, such as massage oils or bath blends, may require higher dilution ratios, but these should still be within safe limits.

Patch Testing

Before applying a diluted essential oil blend to a larger area of the body, it's wise to perform a patch test:

Prepare a small amount of the diluted essential oil blend.

Apply a small drop of the blend to a patch of clean skin (e.g., the inside of the forearm).

Wait for 24-48 hours to observe any adverse reactions, such as redness, itching, or irritation.

Other Safety Considerations

Pregnancy and Nursing: Pregnant and nursing women should exercise caution when using essential oils. Consult with a healthcare professional or aromatherapist for guidance.

Phototoxic Oils: Some essential oils, like citrus oils (e.g., lemon, bergamot), can make the skin more sensitive to sunlight, potentially leading to sunburn. Avoid direct sun exposure after applying phototoxic oils to the skin.

Ingestion: Ingesting essential oils is a controversial practice and should be done with extreme caution, only under the guidance of a qualified aromatherapist or healthcare practitioner.

Storage Considerations

Apart from dilution and application, the safe storage of essential oils is equally crucial to maintain their quality and potency:

Dark Glass Bottles: Essential oils should be stored in dark glass bottles to protect them from light exposure, which can cause them to degrade over time.

Cool, Dry Place: Keep your essential oils in a cool, dry place away from direct sunlight and extreme temperature fluctuations. This helps prevent oxidation and evaporation of volatile compounds.

Childproof Caps: Use childproof caps on essential oil bottles to prevent accidental ingestion or spills, especially if you have children or pets in your household.

Proper Sealing: Ensure that the bottles are tightly sealed after each use to minimize exposure to air, which can lead to oxidation.

Labeling: Properly label your essential oil bottles with the name of the oil, date of purchase, and any specific safety instructions or dilution ratios you've prepared.

Dilution for Specific Applications

While a 2-3% dilution is a common guideline for many applications, certain situations may require different dilution ratios:

Massage Oil: For a massage blend, you can use a higher dilution ratio, typically between 2-5%, depending on the client's preference and skin sensitivity.

Bath: When adding essential oils to a bath, it's best to first dilute them in a carrier oil or bath salts to disperse them evenly in the water and minimize the risk of skin irritation.

Diffusion: In aromatherapy diffusers, undiluted essential oils can be used safely, but it's essential to follow the manufacturer's instructions regarding the number of drops to add.

Hair Care: When using essential oils for hair care, such as in shampoos or conditioners, the dilution ratio can vary but is generally around 1-2%.

Educating Yourself

To use essential oils safely and effectively, consider these educational steps:

Consult Experts: Seek advice from qualified aromatherapists, herbalists, or healthcare professionals who have experience with essential oils.

Reference Books: Invest in reputable books and resources on essential oils and aromatherapy to deepen your knowledge.

Courses and Workshops: Consider enrolling in certified courses or workshops on aromatherapy and essential oil usage. Many institutions offer online and in-person training programs.

Community and Forums: Join online communities or forums of like-minded individuals who share experiences and insights on essential oil use.

Continual Learning: Keep up-to-date with the latest research and developments in the field of aromatherapy and essential oils. Knowledge is continually evolving.

Chapter 19: Blending Essential Oils for Maximum Effect

Creating essential oil blends is both an art and a science, offering a unique way to harness the diverse therapeutic properties of different oils. In this chapter, we'll explore the principles of blending essential oils for maximum effectiveness and various approaches to crafting well-balanced and purpose-driven blends.

The Art and Science of Blending

Blending essential oils involves combining two or more oils to achieve a specific therapeutic or aromatic goal. It's a creative process that requires an understanding of each oil's properties, aroma, and potential synergies.

Selecting Essential Oils

Base, Middle, and Top Notes: Essential oils are often categorized into base, middle, and top notes based on their aroma and volatility. Blends typically include oils from each category to create a harmonious scent profile and therapeutic effect.

Therapeutic Goals: Identify the primary purpose of your blend, whether it's for relaxation, energizing, pain relief, skincare, or emotional support. Select oils known for their relevant properties.

Aroma: Consider the desired aroma profile. Some blends are crafted for their pleasing scents, while others prioritize therapeutic benefits.

Blending Ratios

The blending ratio determines the concentration of each essential oil in the final blend. Common blending ratios include:

Equal Parts (1:1:1): Each oil in the blend is used in equal amounts, creating a balanced profile.

Balanced (1:2:1): This ratio places more emphasis on the middle note, creating depth in the blend.

Harmony (1:2:2): The top and middle notes are doubled in quantity, allowing for a more complex aroma.

Therapeutic (1:5:3): A ratio often used for therapeutic blends, with more emphasis on the base note for grounding and stability.

Blending Techniques

Layering: Start with the base note, followed by the middle and top notes. This method allows for gradual evaporation and a changing aroma over time.

Rolling or Shaking: Roll or shake the blend to mix the oils thoroughly. This is especially useful when creating blends for topical use.

Smelling Strips: Use smelling strips or blotter paper to test and refine your blend's aroma. This helps you make adjustments before finalizing the blend.

Recording and Experimentation

Keep Records: Maintain a journal or digital records of your blend recipes, including the oils used, ratios, and intended purpose. This allows you to replicate successful blends and learn from experiments.

Experiment and Adjust: Don't be afraid to experiment with different oils and ratios. Essential oil blending is an evolving process, and you may discover unique combinations that work best for your needs.

Safety Considerations

Patch Testing: Before applying a new blend to a larger area of the body, always perform a patch test to check for skin sensitivities or allergic reactions.

Dilution: Ensure that your final blend is properly diluted for the intended application. Follow dilution guidelines for safe use on the skin or in diffusers.

Phototoxicity: Be aware of phototoxic essential oils (e.g., citrus oils) that can make the skin sensitive to sunlight. Avoid sun exposure after using phototoxic oils topically.

Storage and Labeling

Dark Glass Bottles: Store your blends in dark glass bottles to protect them from light exposure, which can degrade the oils.

Labeling: Clearly label your blends with their names, ingredients, ratios, and date of creation. Proper labeling ensures you can identify and use them correctly.

One of the most fascinating aspects of essential oil blending is the potential for synergy. Synergy occurs when the combined effects of essential oils are greater than the sum of their individual effects. This means that a well-crafted blend can deliver enhanced therapeutic benefits or a more complex and harmonious aroma than any single oil.

Here are a few key principles to keep in mind for achieving synergy and balance in your blends:

Complementary Properties: Choose oils with complementary therapeutic properties to achieve a specific goal. For example, if you're creating a blend to ease respiratory congestion, consider combining eucalyptus (for its decongestant properties) with lavender (for relaxation).

Harmonious Aroma: The aroma of your blend should be pleasant and balanced. Aim for a blend that doesn't have one overpowering scent but rather a harmonious bouquet of top, middle, and base notes. This can make the blend more enjoyable for personal use and in aromatherapy.

Experimentation: Achieving the perfect blend often involves experimentation. Start with small test batches and adjust the ratios until you achieve the desired effect. The art of blending is about finding what works best for you or your intended audience.

Intuitive Blending

As you gain experience in blending essential oils, you may develop an intuitive sense for which oils work well together and what ratios are most effective. Trust your instincts and creativity when crafting blends, and don't be afraid to step outside established guidelines.

Advanced Blending Techniques

Advanced blending techniques involve using essential oils in layers or using base, middle, and top notes strategically to create more complex and evolving aromas. These techniques require a deeper understanding of each oil's volatility and aroma profile.

Layering: Apply the oils in layers, starting with the base notes, followed by the middle notes, and finally the top notes. This approach allows the blend's scent to evolve over time as each layer gradually evaporates.

Symphony Blending: This technique involves blending several oils within each category (base, middle, and top notes) to create a symphony of scents. It results in a blend with multiple layers and nuances.

Blending for Emotional Well-Being

Blending essential oils for emotional support is a unique and rewarding practice. Aromatherapy can have a profound impact on emotions and mood. Here are some ideas for blending with emotional well-being in mind:

Balancing Blend: Combine oils known for their calming and uplifting properties, such as lavender, bergamot, and ylang-ylang, to create a balanced and harmonizing blend.

Stress Relief: Craft blends that help relieve stress and anxiety. Essential oils like chamomile, frankincense, and clary sage can be soothing and grounding.

Mood Enhancement: Create blends that boost mood and energy. Citrus oils like lemon, orange, and grapefruit are known for their invigorating and mood-lifting effects.

Self-Care Rituals: Design blends to enhance self-care rituals, such as meditation, relaxation, or bedtime routines. These blends can create a soothing and comforting atmosphere.

Blending as a Personal Journey

Remember that blending essential oils is a personal journey. Your preferences, sensitivities, and therapeutic needs will guide your choices and techniques. Embrace the artistry of blending, enjoy the aromatic experiences you create, and continue to explore the vast world of essential oils as you embark on this fragrant and therapeutic journey.

Chapter 20: Aromatherapy: Healing Through Scent

Aromatherapy is an ancient healing practice that utilizes the aromatic properties of essential oils to promote physical, emotional, and mental well-being. In this chapter, we will explore the art and science of aromatherapy, its historical roots, and how it can be used as a powerful tool for holistic healing.

Historical Roots of Aromatherapy

Aromatherapy has deep historical roots that can be traced back thousands of years across various cultures:

Ancient Civilizations: The use of aromatic plants and oils for medicinal, spiritual, and cosmetic purposes was common in civilizations such as Egypt, Greece, Rome, and China.

Ayurveda: In Ayurvedic medicine, an ancient Indian system of healing, aromatic substances played a vital role in promoting balance and harmony within the body and mind.

Traditional Chinese Medicine: Aromatics like frankincense and myrrh were used in Traditional Chinese Medicine to influence the flow of vital energy (Qi) and to treat various health issues.

Middle Ages and Renaissance: During the Middle Ages and Renaissance, herbalism and the use of aromatic oils for therapeutic purposes thrived in Europe.

Modern Aromatherapy: Aromatherapy as we know it today emerged in the early 20th century when French chemist René-Maurice Gattefossé coined the term "aromatherapy" after discovering the healing properties of lavender oil.

Aromatherapy Principles

Aromatherapy is based on several key principles:

Essential Oils: The core of aromatherapy is the use of essential oils, which are extracted from aromatic plant parts. These oils contain the concentrated essence and therapeutic properties of the plants.

Holistic Approach: Aromatherapy considers the whole person, including physical, emotional, and mental aspects. It aims to balance and harmonize these aspects for overall well-being.

Individualization: Aromatherapy recognizes that each person is unique, and treatments should be tailored to individual needs and preferences.

Absorption: Essential oils can be absorbed through the skin, inhalation, or ingestion (with extreme caution and guidance from a qualified practitioner). The chosen method depends on the desired therapeutic effect.

Methods of Application

Aromatherapy offers various methods of application, each suited to specific needs and preferences:

Inhalation: Inhaling the aroma of essential oils can have a direct impact on mood and emotions. Methods include diffusers, steam inhalation, and aromatherapy jewelry.

Topical Application: Essential oils can be diluted in carrier oils and applied to the skin for massage or targeted relief. This method is suitable for addressing physical ailments, such as muscle tension or skin conditions.

Baths: Adding a few drops of essential oils to a bath can create a relaxing and therapeutic experience. The warm water enhances the absorption of the oils through the skin.

Compresses: Warm or cold compresses infused with essential oils can be applied to specific areas of the body to alleviate pain or inflammation.

Internal Use: In some cases, essential oils are used internally under the guidance of a qualified aromatherapist or healthcare professional. However, this method should be approached with extreme caution.

Common Aromatherapy Uses

Aromatherapy can address a wide range of physical and emotional issues:

Stress and Anxiety: Essential oils like lavender, chamomile, and frankincense are known for their calming properties and can help reduce stress and anxiety.

Sleep Disorders: Aromatherapy can promote relaxation and improve sleep quality. Oils like lavender and cedarwood are often used for this purpose.

Pain Relief: Some essential oils, such as peppermint and eucalyptus, have analgesic properties and can be applied topically to alleviate pain.

Skin Care: Essential oils like tea tree, lavender, and rosehip can be used in skincare to address various skin issues, including acne, eczema, and aging.

Respiratory Health: Oils like eucalyptus and peppermint can help relieve congestion and support respiratory health when inhaled.

Emotional Balance: Aromatherapy can influence mood and emotions. Citrus oils like lemon and bergamot are often used for their uplifting effects.

Safety and Precautions

While aromatherapy is generally safe when used correctly, it's essential to exercise caution:

Dilution: Always dilute essential oils in a suitable carrier oil before applying them to the skin to prevent irritation or sensitization.

Phototoxicity: Be aware of phototoxic oils that can make the skin more sensitive to sunlight, and avoid sun exposure after topical use.

Pregnancy and Medical Conditions: Consult with a qualified aromatherapist or healthcare professional, especially if you are pregnant, nursing, or have underlying medical conditions.

Aromatherapy and the Mind-Body Connection

One of the most compelling aspects of aromatherapy is its ability to bridge the gap between the physical and emotional realms. It recognizes the profound connection between scent and emotions, and how the aromatic compounds in essential oils can influence mood, reduce stress, and enhance emotional well-being.

Emotional Release: Aromatherapy can act as a powerful tool for emotional release and processing. Certain essential oils, such as rose or jasmine, are known for their ability to evoke feelings of joy, love, and comfort.

Stress Reduction: The soothing scents of lavender, chamomile, and geranium can help reduce stress and anxiety. Inhaling these oils or using them in a diffuser can create a calming atmosphere.

Mood Elevation: Aromatherapy can uplift and elevate mood. Citrus oils like lemon, orange, and grapefruit are popular choices for their invigorating and cheerful aromas.

The Role of Essential Oils

Essential oils are the heart and soul of aromatherapy. These concentrated extracts capture the essence of plants and offer a diverse range of therapeutic properties:

Chemical Complexity: Essential oils are composed of a complex mixture of natural chemicals, including terpenes, phenols, esters, and more. Each chemical component contributes to the oil's unique aroma and therapeutic effects.

Individual Variability: Just as people have unique preferences and sensitivities, essential oils have individual profiles. What works well for one person may not have the same effect on another. A skilled aromatherapist can help tailor treatments to individual needs.

Scent Memory: Scent has a remarkable ability to evoke memories and emotions. Aromatherapists often tap into this phenomenon to facilitate emotional healing and well-being.

Customized Aromatherapy Blends

Aromatherapists and individuals alike often create customized essential oil blends tailored to specific needs:

Personalized Formulas: Aromatherapists work closely with clients to understand their physical and emotional concerns, crafting unique blends that address those specific issues.

DIY Blending: Enthusiasts of aromatherapy can experiment with creating their own blends for various purposes, from relaxation to skincare. This hands-on approach allows for a deeper connection with the oils and their effects.

Aromatherapy in Modern Healthcare

Aromatherapy is increasingly integrated into modern healthcare settings, including hospitals, hospices, and wellness centers:

Palliative Care: Aromatherapy is used in palliative care to enhance the quality of life for individuals with terminal illnesses, providing comfort and relief.

Stress Reduction: Healthcare professionals use aromatherapy to help reduce stress and anxiety among patients, promoting a sense of calm and relaxation.

Pain Management: Essential oils like lavender and peppermint are applied topically or inhaled to alleviate pain and discomfort in clinical settings.

Complementary Care: Aromatherapy is often used as a complementary therapy alongside conventional medical treatments, promoting holistic well-being.

Aromatherapy at Home

Aromatherapy need not be confined to clinical settings. Many individuals incorporate it into their daily lives at home:

Diffusers: Diffusers are popular devices that disperse essential oils into the air. They can create a calming ambiance or provide an invigorating boost.

Topical Applications: Essential oil blends diluted in carrier oils can be applied during self-massage, added to bathwater, or used in skincare routines.

Meditation and Yoga: Aromatherapy is frequently integrated into meditation and yoga practices to enhance relaxation and mindfulness.

Natural Cleaning: Some people use essential oils for natural cleaning solutions, harnessing their antibacterial and antifungal properties.

5. Infusions Unveiled: Making Potent Herbal Drinks for Wellness

Chapter 21: Basics of Herbal Infusions and Decoctions

Herbal infusions and decoctions are fundamental techniques in herbal medicine for extracting the therapeutic properties of plants. In this chapter, we will delve into the principles of these herbal preparations, how to make them, and their various uses for health and well-being.

Understanding Herbal Infusions and Decoctions

Herbal infusions and decoctions are simple yet effective methods for preparing medicinal teas from herbs, roots, leaves, and other plant materials. They are distinguished by their preparation techniques and the parts of the plant used:

Herbal Infusions: An infusion is made by steeping the more delicate parts of a plant, such as leaves, flowers, and aerial parts, in hot water. This method is suitable for extracting volatile compounds, vitamins, and minerals.

Herbal Decoctions: A decoction involves boiling tougher plant materials like roots, bark, seeds, or woody stems in water to extract their therapeutic constituents. Decoctions are used when the active compounds require longer and more vigorous extraction.

Materials Needed

To make herbal infusions and decoctions, you will need the following materials:

Dried or Fresh Herbs: The herbs or plant parts you intend to use for the infusion or decoction.

Water: Fresh, filtered water is best to avoid contaminants that may affect the quality of the preparation.

A Pot or Teapot: Use a clean, non-reactive pot or teapot made of materials like glass, stainless steel, or ceramic.

Strainer: To separate the liquid from the plant material.

Making Herbal Infusions

Here's a step-by-step guide to making herbal infusions:

Boil Water: Bring water to a boil. The amount of water depends on how strong you want your infusion and the specific herb being used.

Place Herbs in a Container: Place the desired amount of dried or fresh herbs in a clean container. Usually, 1-2 teaspoons of dried herbs or 1-2 tablespoons of fresh herbs per cup of water is a good starting point.

Pour Hot Water: Pour the boiling water over the herbs in the container.

Cover and Steep: Cover the container with a lid or plate to trap the volatile compounds, and let the herbs steep for the recommended time (usually 5-15 minutes). Steeping time may vary depending on the herb.

Strain and Serve: After steeping, strain the liquid into a cup, leaving behind the plant material. You can sweeten the infusion with honey, if desired.

Making Herbal Decoctions

Here's how to make herbal decoctions:

Boil Water: Bring water to a boil. Use approximately 1 ounce (30 grams) of plant material for every quart (liter) of water.

Chop or Crush Plant Material: If you're using tough plant materials like roots or bark, chop or crush them into smaller pieces to increase the surface area for extraction.

Add Herbs to Boiling Water: Place the chopped or crushed herbs into the boiling water.

Simmer: Reduce the heat to a gentle simmer and allow the herbs to simmer for 20-30 minutes or longer, depending on the plant material and desired strength.

Strain and Serve: After simmering, strain the decoction to remove the plant material, and serve it while still warm.

Uses of Infusions and Decoctions

Herbal infusions and decoctions have a wide range of applications:

Internal Use: They can be consumed as teas for various health purposes, such as relaxation, digestion, immune support, or as remedies for specific ailments.

External Use: Infusions and decoctions can be used externally for purposes like skin rinses, compresses, and hair treatments.

Hydration: They serve as a pleasant and hydrating way to consume herbal medicine.

Blending: Infusions and decoctions can be used as a base for creating more complex herbal formulations, such as herbal syrups or tinctures.

Customization and Herb Selection

The effectiveness of herbal infusions and decoctions largely depends on the selection of herbs and the customization of your preparations:

Choosing Herbs: Different herbs offer various therapeutic benefits. Research and select herbs that address your specific health concerns or provide the desired flavor experience. For example, peppermint and ginger are commonly used for digestive issues, while chamomile and valerian are known for their calming properties.

Mixing Herbs: Don't hesitate to mix different herbs to create unique blends tailored to your needs or preferences. Blending herbs can enhance both the flavor and therapeutic effects of your infusion or decoction.

Experimentation: Herbal medicine is as much an art as it is a science. Experiment with different herb combinations and infusion or decoction strengths to find what works best for you. Keep records of your recipes and their effects.

Dosage and Duration

To get the most out of your herbal infusions and decoctions, consider these factors:

Dosage: The amount of herbs you use and the strength of your infusion or decoction can vary depending on your goals. For mild daily support, a standard cup of herbal tea made with 1-2 teaspoons of dried herbs is often sufficient. For acute issues or stronger effects, you may increase the herb-to-water ratio.

Frequency: Determine how often you will consume the herbal preparation. Some infusions or decoctions can be enjoyed daily for general well-being, while others may be used as needed for specific health concerns.

Duration: Herbal treatments can vary in duration. Some herbal regimens are short-term, lasting a few days or weeks, while others may be used as ongoing support for chronic conditions. Consult with a qualified herbalist or healthcare provider for guidance on the appropriate dosage and duration for your specific situation.

Storage and Freshness

To maintain the freshness and potency of your herbal infusions and decoctions:

Storage: Store any leftover herbal liquid in a clean glass container in the refrigerator for up to 48 hours. Avoid storing it at room temperature, as it can spoil.

Labeling: Label your herbal preparations with the name of the herbs used, the date of preparation, and any specific instructions or precautions.

Safety Considerations

While herbal infusions and decoctions are generally safe, it's essential to be aware of potential interactions, allergies, and contraindications, especially if you are pregnant, nursing, or taking medications. Consult with a qualified herbalist or healthcare provider if you have concerns about using specific herbs.

Chapter 22: Choosing the Right Herbs for Infusions

Selecting the appropriate herbs for infusions is a crucial step in creating herbal teas that are not only flavorful but also effective for various health and wellness purposes. In this chapter, we will explore the key factors to consider when choosing herbs for your infusions and delve into some popular herbal options.

Factors to Consider When Choosing Herbs

Intended Purpose: The first consideration is the specific goal you want to achieve with your herbal infusion. Different herbs have distinct therapeutic properties, so you should choose herbs that align with your intended purpose. For instance:

Digestive Health: If you want to support digestion, herbs like peppermint, ginger, or fennel are excellent choices.

Relaxation and Sleep: For relaxation and sleep aid, consider herbs like chamomile, lavender, or valerian.

Immune Support: To boost your immune system, try herbs such as echinacea, elderberry, or astragalus.

Flavor Profile: The flavor of the herbs should complement your taste preferences. Some herbs have strong, bold flavors, while others are milder and more delicate. Consider what tastes you enjoy and choose herbs accordingly.

Minty: Peppermint and spearmint add a refreshing, invigorating flavor.

Floral: Chamomile and rose petals provide a gentle, floral aroma and taste.

Earthy: Nettles and dandelion root offer earthy, slightly bitter notes.

Citrusy: Lemongrass and lemon balm provide a zesty, citrus-like taste.

Safety and Allergies: Be aware of any allergies or sensitivities you or your intended consumers may have. Some herbs may cause allergic reactions or interact with medications, so it's crucial to do your research or consult with a healthcare professional if you have concerns.

Herb Quality: Choose high-quality, organic herbs whenever possible. Organic herbs are grown without synthetic pesticides or herbicides, which can be present in conventionally grown herbs.

Fresh vs. Dried: Both fresh and dried herbs can be used for infusions. Dried herbs have a longer shelf life and are readily available, making them a convenient choice. Fresh herbs, on the other hand, provide a more vibrant and immediate flavor but may not be as accessible year-round.

Single Herbs vs. Blends: You can use single herbs or create your own herbal blends. Single herbs allow you to experience the specific properties of one plant, while blends can offer a broader spectrum of flavors and benefits.

Popular Herbs for Infusions

Here are some popular herbs for infusions and their general uses:

Chamomile (Matricaria chamomilla):

Flavor: Gentle, apple-like flavor.

Uses: Promotes relaxation, eases digestive discomfort, supports sleep.

Peppermint (Mentha x piperita):

Flavor: Refreshing and minty.

Uses: Aids digestion, relieves headaches, invigorates.

Lavender (Lavandula angustifolia):

Flavor: Floral and soothing.

Uses: Calms the mind, promotes relaxation, eases anxiety.

Ginger (Zingiber officinale):

Flavor: Spicy and warming.

Uses: Aids digestion, reduces nausea, supports circulation.

Echinacea (Echinacea purpurea):

Flavor: Earthy and slightly bitter.

Uses: Boosts immune function, reduces the severity of cold symptoms.

Lemon Balm (Melissa officinalis):

Flavor: Citrusy and uplifting.

Uses: Relieves stress, eases indigestion, promotes a positive mood.

Nettle (Urtica dioica):

Flavor: Earthy and green.

Uses: Supports allergies, provides nutrients, aids in detoxification.

Rose Hips (Rosa spp.):

Flavor: Tart and fruity.

Uses: Rich in vitamin C, supports the immune system, enhances skin health.

Experimentation and Personalization

Ultimately, choosing the right herbs for your infusions is a personal journey. Don't hesitate to experiment with different herbs, ratios, and blends to find what resonates with your taste buds and aligns with your wellness goals. Whether you're seeking relaxation, digestive support, or an immune boost, there is a world of herbal possibilities to explore in crafting flavorful and beneficial infusions.

Herbs for Specific Health Needs

To help you further navigate the world of herbal infusions, let's explore some herbs that are renowned for their specific health benefits:

Elderberry (Sambucus spp.):

Flavor: Sweet and fruity.

Uses: Supports the immune system, particularly during cold and flu season. It's a popular choice for immune-boosting infusions and syrups.

Dandelion Root (Taraxacum officinale):

Flavor: Earthy and slightly bitter.

Uses: Known for its detoxifying properties, dandelion root infusions can support liver health and aid digestion. It's often used as a coffee substitute when roasted.

Valerian (Valeriana officinalis):

Flavor: Earthy and pungent.

Uses: Valerian root infusions are famous for their calming and sedative effects. They can help with anxiety, insomnia, and relaxation.

Hibiscus (Hibiscus sabdariffa):

Flavor: Tart and fruity.

Uses: Hibiscus infusions are rich in antioxidants and vitamin C. They can support cardiovascular health and provide a refreshing, tangy beverage.

Raspberry Leaf (Rubus idaeus):

Flavor: Mild and slightly astringent.

Uses: Raspberry leaf infusions are often consumed during pregnancy to support uterine health and ease menstrual discomfort. They can also be enjoyed for their pleasant taste.

Thyme (Thymus vulgaris):

Flavor: Herbaceous and slightly savory.

Uses: Thyme infusions can provide respiratory support and help alleviate coughs and congestion. Thyme is often used in herbal blends for respiratory health.

Licorice Root (Glycyrrhiza glabra):

Flavor: Sweet and naturally sugary.

Uses: Licorice root infusions can soothe the throat and provide relief from coughs and colds. They also have mild anti-inflammatory properties.

Turmeric (Curcuma longa):

Flavor: Earthy and slightly spicy.

Uses: Turmeric root infusions are packed with anti-inflammatory and antioxidant compounds. They can support joint health and overall well-being.

Safety and Precautions

While herbal infusions are generally safe, it's crucial to be aware of any potential contraindications or interactions:

Pregnancy and Nursing: Some herbs are not recommended during pregnancy or while breastfeeding. Consult with a qualified herbalist or healthcare provider for guidance.

Medications: Certain herbs can interact with medications. If you are taking prescription drugs, check for potential herb-drug interactions.

Allergies: Be mindful of any allergies to herbs or related plants. Even mild allergic reactions can be unpleasant.

Dosage: Stick to recommended dosages and avoid excessive consumption, especially with potent herbs.

Quality: Ensure you are using high-quality herbs from reputable sources to minimize the risk of contaminants.

Chapter 23: Cold Infusions: Benefits and Methods

Cold infusions offer a refreshing and unique way to extract the flavors and benefits of herbs without the use of heat. In this chapter, we will explore the benefits of cold infusions, when to use them, and methods for preparing these herbal delights.

Understanding Cold Infusions

Cold infusions, also known as cold brews, are herbal preparations that extract the goodness of herbs using cold or room-temperature water instead of hot water. This gentle method is particularly suitable for herbs that are sensitive to heat or for those times when you prefer a cooler, thirst-quenching herbal drink.

Benefits of Cold Infusions

Preservation of Volatile Compounds: Cold infusions are excellent for preserving the volatile compounds in herbs, such as essential oils, which can be lost through the evaporation that occurs with hot infusions.

Milder Flavor Profile: Cold infusions tend to yield milder, less bitter flavors compared to hot infusions or decoctions. This makes them an ideal choice for herbs with delicate or subtle flavors.

Refreshment: Cold infusions are perfect for hot summer days, providing a cooling and hydrating beverage that can be enjoyed over ice.

Minimal Oxidation: The cold extraction process minimizes oxidation, preserving the freshness and potency of the herbs.

When to Use Cold Infusions

Warm Weather: Cold infusions are especially enjoyable during warm weather when you're seeking a refreshing and hydrating herbal drink.

Delicate Herbs: Herbs that lose their delicate flavors and aromas when exposed to heat, such as mint or some floral herbs, are well-suited for cold infusions.

Children and Seniors: Cold infusions are a safer option for children and seniors who may be at risk of burning themselves with hot liquids.

Preserving Nutrients: If you want to preserve the maximum nutritional content of herbs, cold infusions are a good choice.

Methods for Making Cold Infusions

Making a cold infusion is a straightforward process:

Choose Your Herbs: Select the herbs you want to use. Fresh or dried herbs can be used for cold infusions.

Measure: Determine the amount of herbs you want to use. Generally, 1-2 teaspoons of dried herbs or 1-2 tablespoons of fresh herbs per cup of water is a good starting point.

Combine Herbs and Water: Place the herbs in a clean glass container, such as a jar or pitcher. Add cold or room-temperature filtered water to cover the herbs.

Steep: Cover the container and let the herbs steep for an extended period, typically 4-8 hours or overnight. This extended steeping time allows for gentle extraction without heat.

Strain: After steeping, strain the liquid to remove the herbs. You can use a fine-mesh strainer or a piece of cheesecloth.

Flavor Enhancements: If desired, you can add flavor enhancements like lemon slices, honey, or a touch of fruit juice to your cold infusion for added taste.

Serve: Your cold infusion is ready to be served over ice or enjoyed as is.

Popular Herbs for Cold Infusions

While many herbs can be used for cold infusions, some are particularly well-suited for this method:

Mint (Mentha spp.):

Flavor: Refreshing and cooling.

Uses: Ideal for soothing digestion and providing a crisp, invigorating taste.

Cucumber (Cucumis sativus):

Flavor: Mild and subtly earthy.

Uses: Known for its hydration benefits, cucumber-infused water is a popular choice in hot weather.

Lemon Balm (Melissa officinalis):

Flavor: Citrusy and uplifting.

Uses: Offers a lemony zing and supports relaxation and mood.

Fruit Blends:

Flavor: Fruity and sweet.

Uses: Combining fruits like berries, oranges, or apples with herbs creates a delightful and flavorful cold infusion.

Lavender (Lavandula angustifolia):

Flavor: Floral and soothing.

Uses: Lavender-infused water provides a calming and aromatic experience.

Experiment and Enjoy

Cold infusions open up a world of possibilities for creating refreshing herbal drinks. By exploring different herbs and flavor combinations, you can craft unique and thirst-quenching beverages that not only delight your taste buds but also provide the potential health benefits of the herbs. Whether you're sipping a cool mint infusion on a hot day or experimenting with fruit and herb blends, cold infusions offer a versatile and enjoyable way to integrate herbs into your daily life.

Enhancing Cold Infusions

While the basic method of making cold infusions involves steeping herbs in cold water, you can elevate your creations with additional enhancements and creative ideas:

Fruit Additions: Incorporate slices of fresh fruit like strawberries, oranges, or berries into your cold infusion for a burst of natural sweetness and flavor. This adds a visually appealing touch and enhances the taste.

Herb Combinations: Experiment with combining different herbs to create complex flavor profiles. For instance, a blend of mint and lemon balm can result in a refreshing and soothing infusion.

Honey or Sweeteners: If you prefer your cold infusion on the sweeter side, consider adding a touch of honey, agave nectar, or stevia. Stir the sweetener into your cold infusion until it's fully dissolved.

Citrus Zest: Grate the zest of lemons, limes, or oranges into your cold infusion for a citrusy twist. The zest adds a bright and aromatic dimension to the drink.

Bubbly Cold Infusions: Transform your cold infusion into a sparkling beverage by mixing it with carbonated water or soda. This effervescent twist can make for a delightful and fizzy drink.

Garnishes: Elevate the presentation of your cold infusion by garnishing each glass with a sprig of fresh herbs, a twist of citrus peel, or edible flowers.

Cold Infusion Storage

Proper storage ensures the freshness and safety of your cold infusions:

Refrigeration: Store your cold infusion in the refrigerator to prevent spoilage. Consume it within 24-48 hours for the best quality.

Glass Containers: Use glass containers with tight-sealing lids to store your infusions. Glass is non-reactive and won't affect the taste of your infusion.

Avoid Direct Sunlight: Keep your infusion away from direct sunlight, as sunlight can cause degradation of certain compounds and affect the taste.

Cold Infusions for Health and Well-Being

In addition to being a delightful and refreshing beverage, cold infusions can offer health benefits depending on the herbs you use:

Hydration: Staying hydrated is crucial for overall well-being, and cold infusions are an enticing way to increase your water intake.

Digestive Support: Herbs like mint, ginger, and fennel in cold infusions can aid digestion, making them a pleasant post-meal option.

Stress Relief: Herbs like lemon balm and lavender in cold infusions can have calming properties, promoting relaxation and stress relief.

Antioxidant Boost: Many herbs used in cold infusions are rich in antioxidants, which can help protect cells from oxidative damage.

Vitamin Intake: Some herbs and fruits in cold infusions provide essential vitamins and minerals, contributing to your daily nutrient intake.

Chapter 24: Long Infusions for Deep Healing

Long infusions, also known as extended or overnight infusions, are a unique herbal preparation method that involves steeping herbs for an extended period, typically 4-8 hours or even overnight. In this chapter, we will explore the benefits of long infusions, how to make them, and some herbs commonly used in this method.

Understanding Long Infusions

Long infusions are a gentle and time-intensive way of extracting the full range of therapeutic compounds from herbs. Unlike quick infusions, which are steeped for a short time in hot water, long infusions allow for a slow and thorough extraction of herbal goodness using cold or room-temperature water. This method is particularly suitable for herbs that benefit from prolonged contact with water to release their medicinal properties fully.

Benefits of Long Infusions

Full Spectrum Extraction: Long infusions capture a broader range of plant constituents, including volatile oils, vitamins, minerals, and complex phytochemicals. This results in a more comprehensive and potent herbal extract.

Nutrient Retention: The extended steeping process preserves the nutritional value of herbs, making long infusions an excellent way to obtain vitamins, minerals, and other nutrients from plants.

Delicate Herbs: Herbs with delicate flavors and therapeutic compounds that are easily destroyed by heat, such as certain aromatic herbs and leafy greens, are well-suited for long infusions.

Deep Healing: Long infusions are often used for deep healing, addressing chronic conditions, and providing long-term support to the body.

How to Make Long Infusions

Creating a long infusion involves the following steps:

Choose Your Herbs: Select the herbs you want to use. Both dried and fresh herbs can be used for long infusions.

Measure: Determine the amount of herbs you want to use. Generally, 1-2 teaspoons of dried herbs or 1-

2 tablespoons of fresh herbs per cup of water is a good starting point.

Combine Herbs and Water: Place the herbs in a clean glass container, such as a jar or pitcher. Add cold or room-temperature filtered water to cover the herbs.

Steep for an Extended Period: Cover the container and let the herbs steep for an extended period. The duration can vary but often ranges from 4-8 hours or overnight. You can place the container in the refrigerator during this time to prevent spoilage.

Strain: After the extended steeping period, strain the liquid to remove the herbs. You can use a fine-mesh strainer or a piece of cheesecloth.

Flavor Enhancements: If desired, you can add flavor enhancements like a squeeze of lemon, a drizzle of honey, or a touch of fruit juice to your long infusion.

Serve: Your long infusion is ready to be served. It can be consumed at room temperature or chilled.

Herbs Commonly Used in Long Infusions

While a wide range of herbs can be used for long infusions, some are particularly well-suited for this method:

Nettle (Urtica dioica):

Benefits: Nettle is rich in vitamins, minerals, and antioxidants. It's often used for overall well-being, including support for the skin, hair, and nails.

Oatstraw (Avena sativa):

Benefits: Oatstraw is known for its nourishing and calming properties. It can promote relaxation and support the nervous system.

Red Clover (Trifolium pratense):

Benefits: Red clover is used for its phytoestrogen content and is believed to support hormone balance. It's often used for menopausal symptoms.

Raspberry Leaf (Rubus idaeus):

Benefits: Raspberry leaf is traditionally used to support uterine health and is commonly consumed during pregnancy.

Linden (Tilia spp.):

Benefits: Linden flowers are known for their calming and soothing properties. They can be used to relax and ease tension.

Dandelion Leaf (Taraxacum officinale):

Benefits: Dandelion leaf is rich in vitamins and minerals and is often used for its diuretic and detoxifying properties.

Astragalus (Astragalus membranaceus):

Benefits: Astragalus is valued for its immune-supportive properties. It's commonly used during the cold and flu season.

Deep Healing with Long Infusions

Long infusions are ideal for deep healing and addressing chronic conditions because they provide a sustained release of herbal compounds over an extended period. When incorporating long infusions into your wellness routine, consider the following:

Consistency: For deep healing, it's essential to be consistent with your long infusion regimen. Drinking a cup daily or as recommended by an herbalist can provide ongoing support.

Patience: Long-term benefits often require patience. Allow time for the herbs to work their magic, and you may start noticing improvements in your overall well-being.

Monitoring: Keep track of any changes or improvements in your health and consult with a qualified herbalist or healthcare provider for guidance on long-term use.

Exploring Herbal Synergy in Long Infusions

One of the remarkable aspects of long infusions is their ability to capture the synergy between multiple herbs. You can create blends of herbs that complement each other's actions, resulting in a potent and well-rounded infusion. Here are a few examples of herb combinations for long infusions:

Nourishing Blend: Combine oatstraw, nettle, and red clover for a nourishing infusion that supports overall well-being. Oatstraw calms the nerves, nettle provides essential nutrients, and red clover offers hormonal support.

Immune Boost: Create an immune-boosting infusion by blending astragalus, echinacea, and elderberry. Astragalus enhances immune function, echinacea provides immune stimulation, and elderberry offers antiviral properties.

Digestive Support: Combine peppermint, fennel, and ginger for a soothing and digestive-friendly infusion. Peppermint relaxes the digestive tract, fennel eases bloating, and ginger aids digestion.

Hormonal Harmony: Craft an infusion with red raspberry leaf, dong quai, and vitex for hormonal balance. Red raspberry leaf supports uterine health, dong quai balances hormones, and vitex aids in regulating the menstrual cycle.

Stress Relief: Create a calming blend with chamomile, lemon balm, and linden. Chamomile relaxes, lemon balm eases tension, and linden soothes the nervous system.

Adapting Long Infusions to Your Needs

Long infusions are versatile and adaptable to your specific health needs and taste preferences:

Flavor Enhancement: While long infusions can be enjoyed as is, you can also add flavor enhancements like a squeeze of lemon, a drizzle of honey, or a touch of herbal sweeteners like stevia or licorice root.

Cold or Warm: Long infusions can be consumed cold, similar to cold infusions, or gently heated for a warm and comforting beverage during cooler months.

Variation in Strength: The strength of your long infusion can be adjusted by altering the herb-to-water ratio or the steeping time. Experiment to find the right balance for your taste and needs.

Daily Ritual: Incorporating long infusions into your daily routine can become a soothing and mindful ritual. Whether you enjoy them in the morning to start your day or in the evening to unwind, they can offer a moment of self-care.

Consulting an Herbalist: If you have specific health concerns or are unsure about which herbs to use, consulting with a qualified herbalist can provide personalized guidance and recommendations.

The Journey of Deep Healing

Long infusions offer a holistic approach to deep healing, addressing not only physical but also emotional and spiritual aspects of well-being. As you embark on this journey, you may find that the process of preparing and sipping on your herbal elixirs becomes a meditative practice that connects you more deeply with nature and your inner self.

Remember that deep healing often takes time and patience. Be attentive to your body's responses and consult with a healthcare provider or herbalist when needed. By integrating long infusions into your wellness routine and exploring the myriad possibilities of herbal combinations, you can harness the full potential of nature's healing gifts and embark on a profound journey of well-being and self-discovery.

Chapter 25: Enhancing Flavor and Potency

Enhancing the flavor and potency of herbal preparations is a valuable skill in the world of herbalism. In this chapter, we will explore various methods and strategies to elevate the taste and therapeutic effectiveness of your herbal remedies.

Balancing Flavor and Potency

Before delving into specific techniques, it's crucial to understand the balance between flavor and potency in herbal preparations:

Flavor: The taste of herbal remedies can range from pleasant and mild to strong and bitter. Balancing flavors ensures that your preparations are palatable and enjoyable, making them easier to incorporate into your daily routine.

Potency: Potency refers to the strength and effectiveness of an herbal remedy. It depends on factors such as the quality of herbs used, preparation methods, and dosage. Enhancing potency ensures that your herbal remedies deliver the desired therapeutic benefits.

Enhancing Flavor

Sweeteners: Natural sweeteners like honey, maple syrup, or stevia can be added to herbal preparations to improve taste. These sweeteners not only mask bitterness but also provide additional health benefits. However, use them in moderation to avoid excessive sugar intake.

Citrus: Squeezing a bit of fresh lemon or orange juice into herbal teas or tinctures can impart a refreshing and zesty flavor. Citrus also provides a dose of vitamin C.

Herb Blending: Combining herbs with complementary flavors can create a more balanced taste. For example, adding a hint of mint to a bitter herb infusion can make it more palatable.

Dilution: If an herbal remedy is too strong or bitter, consider diluting it with water or a mild-tasting herbal infusion. This can make it easier to consume while still providing the desired benefits.

Infusion Time: Adjusting the infusion time can impact flavor. Shorter infusion times for some herbs may yield a milder taste, while longer infusions can result in a stronger, more robust flavor.

Enhancing Potency

Quality Herbs: Start with high-quality herbs sourced from reputable suppliers. The potency of herbal remedies begins with the quality of the raw materials.

Proper Storage: Store herbs in a cool, dry place away from direct sunlight. Proper storage helps preserve their potency by preventing degradation.

Correct Dosage: Ensure you are using the recommended dosage for each herb and remedy. Using too little may not yield the desired effects, while using too much can lead to adverse reactions.

Extraction Methods: Experiment with different extraction methods, such as tinctures, decoctions, or macerations, to extract specific compounds and enhance potency.

Combining Herbs: Creating herbal blends that target specific health concerns can increase potency. Some herbs work synergistically when combined, enhancing their overall effectiveness.

Fresh vs. Dried: In some cases, using fresh herbs instead of dried ones can result in more potent remedies, as fresh herbs may contain higher concentrations of active compounds.

Alcohol-Based Tinctures: Alcohol-based tinctures are known for their ability to extract a wide range of compounds from herbs, making them a potent option. However, alcohol-free alternatives are available for those who prefer them.

Safety and Monitoring

When enhancing the flavor and potency of herbal remedies, it's essential to maintain safety and monitor your body's responses:

Start Slowly: When trying a new herbal remedy or increasing the dosage, start with a small amount to gauge your body's reaction.

Monitor Effects: Pay attention to how your body responds to herbal remedies. If you experience any adverse effects or discomfort, discontinue use and seek guidance from a healthcare provider.

Consult a Professional: For complex health issues or when using potent herbs, consult a qualified herbalist or healthcare provider. They can provide personalized guidance and ensure safety.

Synergy in Herbal Combinations

One powerful way to enhance both flavor and potency in herbal preparations is by harnessing the synergy that exists between different herbs. When carefully combined, herbs can complement each other, intensifying their therapeutic effects while often improving the overall taste. Here are some examples of herbal combinations that can amplify both flavor and potency:

Digestive Blend: Combining herbs like ginger, fennel, and peppermint can create a potent digestive blend. Not only do these herbs taste pleasant together, but they also work synergistically to ease indigestion, reduce bloating, and soothe an upset stomach.

Immune-Boosting Elixir: A blend of echinacea, elderberry, and astragalus can enhance the immune-boosting properties of each herb. This combination not only strengthens the immune system but can also yield a rich, berry-like flavor.

Relaxation and Sleep Support: A combination of chamomile, lemon balm, and passionflower can create a calming and sleep-inducing infusion. These herbs work together to relax the nervous system, reduce anxiety, and promote restful sleep while delivering a gentle and soothing taste.

Allergy Relief: Herbs like nettle, quercetin-rich plantain, and eyebright can be blended to combat seasonal allergies. This combination can provide relief from allergy symptoms and create a mildly earthy and slightly sweet infusion.

Women's Health: A blend of red raspberry leaf, dong quai, and vitex can support women's reproductive health. These herbs complement each other in regulating hormones and addressing menstrual concerns while producing a balanced, slightly herbal flavor.

Customization and Experimentation

One of the beauties of herbalism is the freedom to customize and experiment with herbal combinations. You can adjust the ratios of herbs to create a flavor profile that suits your palate while maximizing the therapeutic benefits. Here are some additional tips:

Start with a Base: Choose a primary herb that addresses your specific health concern or desired flavor. Then, add complementary herbs to enhance its effects or taste.

Keep Records: As you experiment with herbal blends, keep a journal to record the ratios and combinations you find most enjoyable and effective. This can be a valuable reference for future use.

Small Batches: When experimenting with new combinations, start with small batches to prevent wastage in case the blend doesn't suit your taste.

Rotate Herbs: Consider rotating the herbs you use over time to prevent your body from developing a tolerance to any one herb. This approach can also provide a variety of flavors and therapeutic benefits.

Final Thoughts

Enhancing the flavor and potency of herbal remedies is a rewarding journey of exploration and self-discovery. By balancing sweetness, acidity, and bitterness, you can create herbal preparations that are not only enjoyable to consume but also deeply beneficial for your health. Additionally, understanding the synergy between different herbs allows you to craft custom blends that amplify the therapeutic effects and flavor profiles, offering a holistic approach to well-being.

As you continue your herbal journey, remember that herbalism is both an art and a science. Don't hesitate to seek guidance from experienced herbalists or healthcare providers, especially when working with potent or unfamiliar herbs. With curiosity and care, you can unlock the full potential of herbs and enhance your overall health and vitality naturally.

6. The Healing Power of Teas: From Leaf to Cup

Chapter 26: A Brief History of Tea as Medicine

Tea has a rich history as a medicinal beverage that dates back thousands of years. In this chapter, we will delve into the origins, evolution, and therapeutic traditions surrounding tea.

The Origins of Tea as Medicine

The story of tea as medicine begins in ancient China, where legend has it that Emperor Shen Nong, a mythical figure in Chinese culture, discovered tea around 2737 BCE. According to the legend, while boiling water under a tea tree, some tea leaves accidentally fell into his pot. He tasted the resulting infusion and found it refreshing and invigorating. This marked the beginning of tea's journey as a beverage and a medicine.

Early Medicinal Uses of Tea

In its early history, tea was primarily valued for its medicinal properties. Chinese herbalists began to explore its potential benefits and categorized it as a medicinal herb. Tea was used to treat a wide range of ailments, from digestive disorders to headaches and fatigue.

The use of tea for its medicinal properties spread to other parts of Asia, including Japan, Korea, and Tibet. In these regions, traditional systems of medicine incorporated tea into their healing practices. For example, in traditional Japanese Kampo medicine, certain types of tea were prescribed to balance the body's vital energies or treat specific health issues.

Tea and Chinese Traditional Medicine

In traditional Chinese medicine (TCM), tea is classified into different categories based on its processing and properties. The two most well-known categories are green tea (lu cha) and black tea (hong cha). Each type of tea was believed to have unique effects on the body:

Green Tea (Lu Cha): Green tea was considered cooling and was often used to clear heat, promote digestion, and soothe the mind. It was also believed to have detoxifying properties.

Black Tea (Hong Cha): Black tea, which was fermented or oxidized, was considered warming and invigorating. It was used to strengthen the digestive system, increase alertness, and improve circulation.

Tea was often prescribed in TCM formulations to enhance the effects of other herbs or to mitigate any potential side effects. For example, green tea might be combined with herbs that clear heat, while black tea might be used alongside warming herbs to treat cold conditions.

Tea on the Silk Road and Beyond

As trade routes expanded along the Silk Road, tea became a valuable commodity and traveled to various parts of the world. Along with the leaves, knowledge of tea's medicinal properties also spread. In India, the traditional system of Ayurveda incorporated tea as an herbal remedy, often adding spices like ginger and cardamom to enhance its therapeutic effects.

The Modern Tea Renaissance

In recent years, there has been a resurgence of interest in the health benefits of tea, particularly in the context of scientific research. Studies have explored the antioxidant properties of tea, its potential to support cardiovascular health, aid in weight management, and even reduce the risk of certain chronic diseases.

Green tea, in particular, has been a focus of scientific research due to its high content of polyphenols, such as catechins, which are known for their antioxidant properties.

The Spread of Tea's Medicinal Influence

As tea's reputation as a medicinal beverage grew, it spread across Asia and beyond. Each region developed its own traditions and variations of tea for therapeutic purposes:

Japan: In Japan, tea took on a deeply cultural and ceremonial significance. Matcha, a finely ground green tea, became a centerpiece of the traditional Japanese tea ceremony. It was believed to promote mental clarity and mindfulness, aligning with Zen Buddhist principles. This practice emphasized the integration of the physical, mental, and spiritual aspects of health.

Korea: Korean traditional medicine, known as Hanbang, also embraced tea as a therapeutic tool. Teas made from herbs like ginseng and jujube were used to tonify the body's vital energy, or Qi, and promote overall health. Korean tea ceremonies, while less formal than the Japanese counterpart, shared the idea of tea as a means of balance and harmony.

Tibet: In Tibet, traditional medicine incorporates a variety of herbal teas, often combined with other natural substances like minerals and animal products. These unique blends are believed to balance the body's three humors and treat specific ailments. Tibetan butter tea, made with tea leaves, yak butter, and salt, is a staple in the region, offering sustenance in the harsh Himalayan climate.

The Role of Tea in Ayurveda and Traditional Indian Medicine

In India, the ancient system of Ayurveda recognized the medicinal properties of tea, known as "Chai" in Hindi. Ayurveda classifies herbs, including tea leaves, based on their tastes (rasa), qualities (guna), and effects on the body (virya). The use of spices like ginger, cardamom, and black pepper in chai is not only for flavor but also to balance the doshas, or individual constitutions, according to Ayurvedic principles.

Tea was seen as a harmonizing beverage that could be tailored to an individual's constitution. For example, adding warming spices to tea might balance excess Vata dosha, which is associated with qualities like coldness and dryness. In contrast, cooling herbs and spices might help alleviate Pitta dosha imbalances linked to heat and acidity.

The Modern Era: Scientific Exploration of Tea's Health Benefits

In recent decades, scientific research has rekindled interest in tea's potential health benefits. The focus has been on the bioactive compounds found in tea, particularly in green tea. These compounds, such as catechins, have been studied for their antioxidant, anti-inflammatory, and potential disease-preventing properties.

Some areas of interest in tea research include:

Antioxidant Effects: Tea's high content of polyphenols, especially in green tea, has garnered attention for its potential to neutralize harmful free radicals and protect cells from oxidative stress.

Cardiovascular Health: Studies have explored the link between tea consumption and reduced risk of heart disease, lower blood pressure, and improved cholesterol profiles.

Weight Management: Certain compounds in tea, like EGCG (Epigallocatechin gallate), have been investigated for their role in promoting weight loss and fat metabolism.

Cancer Prevention: Preliminary research has suggested that tea polyphenols may have anticancer properties, potentially reducing the risk of certain types of cancer.

Chapter 27: Types of Teas and Their Healing Properties

Tea comes in various forms, each with its unique characteristics and potential healing properties. In this chapter, we'll explore some of the most popular types of teas and the health benefits associated with them.

Green Tea

Green tea, made from unoxidized tea leaves, is known for its fresh, grassy flavor and a wide range of potential health benefits:

Antioxidant Power: Green tea is rich in catechins, powerful antioxidants that combat oxidative stress and may reduce the risk of chronic diseases.

Heart Health: Regular consumption of green tea has been linked to improved cardiovascular health, including lower LDL cholesterol and reduced blood pressure.

Weight Management: Some studies suggest that green tea extracts can boost metabolism and aid in weight loss efforts.

Mental Alertness: The moderate caffeine content in green tea, combined with the amino acid L-theanine, may promote mental alertness without the jittery effects of coffee.

Anti-Inflammatory: Green tea's polyphenols have anti-inflammatory properties that may help alleviate various conditions, including arthritis.

Black Tea

Black tea, fully oxidized, has a bold and robust flavor. It also offers several potential health benefits:

Heart Health: Like green tea, black tea may help reduce the risk of heart disease by improving cholesterol levels and supporting healthy blood vessel function.

Digestive Aid: Tannins in black tea may have a soothing effect on the digestive tract, potentially alleviating digestive discomfort.

Energy Boost: The caffeine content in black tea can provide an energy boost and increased mental alertness.

Oral Health: Some studies suggest that the polyphenols in black tea may help prevent the growth of bacteria in the mouth, promoting better oral health.

Herbal Teas

Herbal teas encompass a vast array of infusions made from herbs, spices, flowers, and fruits. Each herbal tea has its own unique flavor and potential health benefits:

Chamomile: Chamomile tea is known for its calming properties, making it a popular choice for relaxation and better sleep. It may also help soothe digestive discomfort.

Peppermint: Peppermint tea is refreshing and often used to alleviate digestive issues like bloating, indigestion, and gas.

Ginger: Ginger tea is a warming and spicy option that may help ease nausea, soothe an upset stomach, and reduce inflammation.

Hibiscus: Hibiscus tea is tart and vibrant, packed with antioxidants that may support heart health and lower blood pressure.

Lavender: Lavender tea is fragrant and soothing, often used for stress relief, anxiety reduction, and better sleep.

White Tea

White tea is made from young tea leaves and buds and is minimally processed, preserving its delicate flavor and potential health benefits:

Antioxidant Rich: White tea contains a high concentration of antioxidants, including catechins, which may help protect against oxidative damage.

Skin Health: Some studies suggest that white tea extracts can promote skin health by reducing the risk of UV damage and preventing premature aging.

Weight Management: White tea may have a role in weight management by enhancing the body's ability to break down and utilize fat.

Oolong Tea

Oolong tea falls between green and black tea in terms of oxidation. It has a diverse flavor profile and offers potential health benefits:

Metabolic Support: Oolong tea is often associated with weight management and may help improve metabolism and fat oxidation.

Antioxidants: Like green and white teas, oolong tea contains antioxidants that combat free radicals and support overall health.

Mental Alertness: The caffeine content in oolong tea can provide a mild energy boost and enhance mental alertness.

Pu-erh Tea

Pu-erh tea is a fermented tea from Yunnan province in China and is known for its earthy, aged flavor. It is believed to offer various health benefits:

Digestive Aid: Pu-erh tea is often consumed after heavy meals to aid in digestion and alleviate bloating.

Cholesterol Management: Some studies suggest that pu-erh tea may help reduce LDL cholesterol levels.

Weight Loss: Pu-erh is often marketed as a weight loss tea, with claims that it can help break down fat in the body.

Rooibos Tea

Rooibos tea, also known as red bush tea, is caffeine-free and hails from South Africa. It boasts a sweet, nutty flavor and potential health benefits:

Antioxidant Properties: Rooibos tea is rich in antioxidants, including quercetin and aspalathin, which may combat oxidative stress.

Anti-Inflammatory: It has anti-inflammatory properties and may help reduce inflammation in the body.

Skin Health: Some people use rooibos topically or drink it for its potential benefits in promoting clear and radiant skin.

Matcha Tea

Matcha is a finely ground green tea traditionally used in Japanese tea ceremonies. It offers a unique preparation method and potential health benefits:

Concentration of Nutrients: Matcha is made from shade-grown tea leaves, resulting in higher concentrations of chlorophyll, antioxidants, and L-theanine compared to regular green tea.

Calm Alertness: Matcha provides a calm sense of alertness due to its combination of caffeine and L-theanine.

Detoxification: Some believe that matcha's chlorophyll content aids in detoxification by promoting the elimination of heavy metals and toxins.

Herbal Blends

Herbal blends are a diverse category that combines various herbs, spices, and botanicals for specific health purposes:

Detox Blends: These may include dandelion, milk thistle, and burdock root to support liver health and detoxification.

Immune Support Blends: Combinations of herbs like echinacea, elderberry, and astragalus may strengthen the immune system.

Digestive Blends: Herbal blends with peppermint, ginger, and fennel can soothe digestive discomfort and promote gut health.

Chai Tea

Chai tea, a spiced Indian tea, offers a rich and aromatic experience, and it blends black tea with a mixture of herbs and spices, often including cinnamon, cardamom, ginger, cloves, and black pepper. Here are some of its potential health benefits:

Digestive Aid: The spices in chai, particularly ginger and cardamom, can aid digestion and relieve gastrointestinal discomfort.

Anti-Inflammatory: Many of the spices in chai, such as cinnamon and cloves, have anti-inflammatory properties that may help reduce inflammation in the body.

Warmth and Comfort: Chai's warming spices provide a sense of comfort and coziness, making it a popular choice during cold weather or for relaxation.

Yerba Mate

Yerba mate is a South American herbal tea made from the leaves of the Ilex paraguariensis plant. It has a grassy and earthy flavor and is traditionally consumed from a gourd with a metal straw called a bombilla. Potential health benefits of yerba mate include:

Energy Boost: Yerba mate contains caffeine, which provides an energy boost similar to coffee but without the jitters.

Antioxidant Properties: It is rich in antioxidants, particularly chlorogenic acid and polyphenols, which combat oxidative stress.

Appetite Control: Some people use yerba mate to help control appetite and support weight management.

Mental Alertness: The combination of caffeine and theobromine in yerba mate can enhance mental alertness and focus.

Kombucha

Kombucha is a fermented tea made by fermenting sweetened tea with a culture of yeast and bacteria. It has a tangy and effervescent quality and potential health benefits, including:

Probiotic Support: Kombucha is a source of beneficial probiotics, which can promote a healthy gut microbiome.

Digestive Health: Probiotics in kombucha may help improve digestion and alleviate digestive issues.

Immune Support: A healthy gut is linked to a strong immune system, so kombucha may indirectly support immune function.

Detoxification: Some people believe that kombucha supports the body's natural detoxification processes.

Floral and Exotic Teas

These teas incorporate a wide range of flowers and exotic herbs, each with its unique flavor and potential health benefits:

Jasmine Tea: Jasmine tea, often made by scenting green tea with jasmine blossoms, is aromatic and may have relaxing and stress-relief properties.

Lavender Tea: Lavender tea, with its gentle floral notes, is soothing and can promote relaxation and better sleep.

Rosehip Tea: Rosehips are high in vitamin C, making rosehip tea a potential immune booster and skin health aid.

Elderflower Tea: Elderflower tea is light and fragrant, often used for its potential immune-supporting properties.

Fruit and Berry Teas

Fruit and berry teas are caffeine-free herbal infusions made from dried fruits, berries, and often hibiscus petals. These teas are naturally sweet and can provide various health benefits:

Vitamin C: Many fruit teas, such as hibiscus or rosehip, are rich in vitamin C, which supports the immune system and skin health.

Hydration: Fruit teas are an excellent choice for hydration, offering a flavorful alternative to plain water.

Antioxidants: The fruits and berries in these teas contribute antioxidants that combat oxidative stress.

Detox Teas

Detox teas are typically blends of herbs like dandelion root, milk thistle, and burdock root, which are believed to support the body's natural detoxification processes. While they are often marketed as detox aids, it's essential to use them in moderation and as part of a balanced diet.

Chapter 28: Brewing the Perfect Cup: Techniques and Tips

Brewing the perfect cup of tea is both an art and a science. It involves careful consideration of factors such as water temperature, steeping time, tea quality, and personal preferences. In this chapter, we will explore various techniques and tips to help you master the art of tea brewing.

Choosing the Right Water

The quality of the water you use plays a significant role in the taste of your tea. Here are some considerations:

Freshness: Always use fresh, cold water that has not been sitting in your kettle or container for an extended period. Stale water can taste flat and affect the tea's flavor.

Filtered vs. Tap: Depending on your location, tap water may contain impurities or chlorine that can negatively impact tea taste. Using filtered water or natural spring water is often recommended.

Measuring Tea Leaves

The amount of tea leaves you use directly affects the flavor and strength of your brew. While the exact measurement may vary depending on the type of tea and personal preference, a general guideline is:

One teaspoon of loose tea leaves for every 8 ounces (about 240 ml) of water.

You can adjust this amount to make your tea stronger or milder.

Water Temperature

Water temperature is crucial because it can affect the extraction of flavors and compounds from the tea leaves. Different types of tea require different temperatures:

Green Tea: Heat water to around 175-185°F (80-85°C). Avoid boiling water, as it can make green tea taste bitter.

Black Tea: Use boiling water, typically around 200-212°F (93-100°C). Black tea's robust flavors can withstand higher temperatures.

White Tea: Opt for water around 160-185°F (71-85°C) to preserve the delicate flavors of white tea.

Herbal Tea: Depending on the herbs used, water temperature can vary. Some herbs prefer boiling water, while others are better with slightly cooler water.

Steeping Time

Steeping time is the duration the tea leaves are in contact with hot water. It can vary widely, so be sure to follow the recommendations for your specific tea. Generally:

Green Tea: 1-3 minutes. Oversteeping can lead to bitterness.

Black Tea: 3-5 minutes. Adjust for your preferred strength.

White Tea: 2-5 minutes. Longer steeping can extract more flavors.

Herbal Tea: Varies by the herbs used. Herbal teas often have longer steeping times, but follow the specific guidelines for your blend.

Teapot or Infuser Choice

The vessel you use for steeping can impact the flavor. Choices include:

Teapot: A teapot with a built-in strainer or infuser basket allows tea leaves to expand fully, releasing more flavor.

Tea Ball or Infuser: These are convenient for single servings but may limit the space for tea leaves to unfurl fully.

Gaiwan: A traditional Chinese teapot with no strainer, allowing for full leaf expansion. It's ideal for gongfu-style tea preparation.

Pre-warming the Teapot

Before adding tea leaves and hot water, it's beneficial to pre-warm the teapot by rinsing it with a small amount of hot water. This ensures the teapot is at a similar temperature to the water used for steeping, preventing temperature shock that can affect flavor.

Experiment and Personalize

Brewing the perfect cup of tea is also about personal preference. Experiment with factors like the amount of tea leaves, water temperature, and steeping time to find what suits your taste best. Keep a tea journal to record your preferences and discoveries.

Proper Storage

To maintain the freshness of your tea leaves, store them in an airtight container away from light, moisture, and strong odors. For long-term storage, consider vacuum-sealed bags or containers with airtight seals.

Water Quality Matters

The quality of your water affects the taste of your tea. If tap water has strong odors or tastes, consider using filtered or bottled spring water.

Clean Your Teaware

Regularly clean your teapot, teacups, and other teaware to prevent the buildup of tea residue, which can affect the flavor of your brew. Use a mild, unscented detergent and rinse thoroughly.

Chapter 29: Custom Tea Blends for Specific Ailments

Custom tea blends offer a versatile and natural way to address specific health concerns and ailments. By combining different herbs, spices, and botanicals, you can create personalized teas that target your unique needs. In this chapter, we will explore how to craft custom tea blends for various common ailments.

Digestive Discomfort

Ingredients: Peppermint leaves, ginger root, fennel seeds, chamomile flowers.

Benefits: Peppermint soothes digestive discomfort, ginger reduces nausea, fennel aids digestion, and chamomile calms the stomach.

How to Make: Combine equal parts of each ingredient in a tea infuser or teapot. Steep in hot water for 5-10 minutes.

Stress and Anxiety

Ingredients: Lavender flowers, chamomile flowers, lemon balm leaves, passionflower.

Benefits: Lavender and chamomile promote relaxation, lemon balm reduces stress, and passionflower has calming properties.

How to Make: Mix these ingredients in the desired proportions (more lavender and chamomile for a calming blend, more lemon balm and passionflower for stress reduction). Steep for 5-7 minutes.

Sleep Support

Ingredients: Valerian root, chamomile flowers, lavender flowers, lemon balm leaves.

Benefits: Valerian induces sleep, chamomile and lavender promote relaxation, and lemon balm eases restlessness.

How to Make: Blend the ingredients with more or less valerian depending on your tolerance. Steep for 10-15 minutes for a restful night's sleep.

Immune Boost

Ingredients: Echinacea root, elderberry, rose hips, ginger.

Benefits: Echinacea supports the immune system, elderberry provides antioxidants, rose hips are rich in vitamin C, and ginger offers anti-inflammatory properties.

How to Make: Combine these ingredients, focusing on equal parts of echinacea and elderberry. Steep for 5-7 minutes.

Respiratory Health

Ingredients: Thyme leaves, eucalyptus leaves, licorice root, peppermint leaves.

Benefits: Thyme and eucalyptus support respiratory health, licorice soothes the throat, and peppermint provides a cooling sensation.

How to Make: Blend the ingredients with a stronger emphasis on thyme and eucalyptus. Steep for 7-10 minutes.

Energy and Focus

Ingredients: Ginseng root, green tea leaves, rosemary leaves, ginkgo biloba leaves.

Benefits: Ginseng boosts energy, green tea provides caffeine for alertness, rosemary enhances memory, and ginkgo biloba improves cognitive function.

How to Make: Adjust the proportions based on your desired energy level. Steep for 3-4 minutes.

Menstrual Pain Relief

Ingredients: Cramp bark, raspberry leaf, ginger, chamomile flowers.

Benefits: Cramp bark eases menstrual cramps, raspberry leaf supports the uterus, ginger reduces inflammation, and chamomile offers relaxation.

How to Make: Create a balanced blend with a focus on cramp bark and raspberry leaf. Steep for 7-10 minutes.

Detox and Cleansing

Ingredients: Dandelion root, burdock root, milk thistle seeds, nettle leaves.

Benefits: Dandelion and burdock aid liver detoxification, milk thistle supports liver health, and nettle acts as a diuretic.

How to Make: Combine these ingredients with a focus on dandelion and burdock. Steep for 10-15 minutes.

Joint Pain and Inflammation

Ingredients: Turmeric root, black pepper, ginger, cinnamon.

Benefits: Turmeric reduces inflammation, black pepper enhances turmeric absorption, ginger offers anti-inflammatory properties, and cinnamon adds flavor.

How to Make: Create a blend with a strong emphasis on turmeric. Steep for 7-10 minutes.

Skin Health

Ingredients: Rooibos tea, calendula petals, nettle leaves, chamomile flowers.

Benefits: Rooibos is rich in antioxidants, calendula soothes the skin, nettle provides vitamins, and chamomile calms irritation.

How to Make: Combine these ingredients in equal parts. Steep for 5-7 minutes.

Customizing Your Blends: The key to crafting custom tea blends is experimentation. Start with a base herb or tea, such as green tea or chamomile, and add other ingredients based on their benefits and your taste preferences. Keep notes on the proportions and brewing times that work best for you.

Chapter 30: Tea Rituals for Mind and Body Wellness

Tea rituals have been practiced for centuries in various cultures around the world, not only for their delightful flavors but also for their potential to promote mental and physical well-being. In this chapter, we will explore different tea rituals that can enhance both mind and body wellness.

Japanese Tea Ceremony (Chanoyu)

The Japanese tea ceremony is a highly choreographed ritual centered around matcha, a powdered green tea. It involves specific movements, utensils, and etiquette. The ceremony promotes mindfulness, harmony, and a sense of presence. Here's how it works:

Preparation: The host meticulously prepares matcha tea for each guest, paying close attention to the quality of the tea, water temperature, and the way it's whisked.

Serving: Guests receive the tea with a bow and enjoy it in silence, savoring both the taste and the peaceful atmosphere.

Appreciation: The tea ceremony encourages mindfulness, as participants appreciate the aesthetics of the tearoom, the craftsmanship of the utensils, and the fleeting beauty of the moment.

Chinese Gongfu Tea Ceremony

The Gongfu tea ceremony is a Chinese tradition that emphasizes the art of brewing and serving tea, particularly oolong and pu-erh teas. It involves a series of precise steps:

Warming the Teapot: The ceremony begins by rinsing the teapot and cups with hot water to ensure they are clean and warm.

Tea Preparation: The tea leaves are carefully measured and placed in the teapot. Hot water is poured over the leaves for a few seconds to rinse them, and then a series of short infusions follow.

Serving: The tea is poured into small cups, and participants savor each infusion, appreciating the evolving flavors.

Connection: Gongfu tea ceremonies are often social, fostering connections and conversations as participants share the tea and their thoughts.

British Afternoon Tea

While less formal than some tea ceremonies, British afternoon tea has its own charm and wellness benefits:

Tea Selection: A variety of teas are offered, typically black teas like Earl Grey or Darjeeling. The process of selecting and brewing tea can be a mindful experience.

Scones and Pastries: While indulgent, the tradition of enjoying scones and pastries with tea can promote relaxation and comfort.

Social Connection: Afternoon tea is often a social event, providing an opportunity to connect with friends and loved ones.

Herbal Infusions for Relaxation

Creating your herbal infusion ritual can be a simple yet effective way to relax and unwind:

Selection: Choose calming herbs like chamomile, lavender, or lemon balm.

Steeping: Use a teapot or a cup with an infuser. Pour hot water over the herbs and let them steep for the recommended time.

Mindfulness: As you sip your herbal infusion, focus on the flavors and sensations. Let go of worries and stress.

Tea Meditation

Tea meditation is a mindfulness practice that can be incorporated into your daily routine:

Select a Special Tea: Choose a tea that you enjoy and find calming, such as green tea or a herbal blend.

Mindful Brewing: Pay attention to every step of the tea-making process, from boiling the water to steeping the tea.

Sip Mindfully: As you sip your tea, be fully present in the moment. Focus on the taste, aroma, and how it makes you feel.

Breathe: Take deep breaths between sips to enhance relaxation and mindfulness.

Herbal Foot Baths

Herbal foot baths are a soothing way to relax and promote wellness:

Ingredients: Add herbs like chamomile, lavender, or rosemary to a basin of warm water.

Soak: Soak your feet in the herbal bath for 15-20 minutes.

Relax: While soaking, focus on deep breathing and releasing tension from your body.

Tea and Journaling

Pairing tea with journaling can be a therapeutic practice:

Selection: Choose a tea that aligns with your intention—whether it's relaxation, inspiration, or focus.

Mindful Sipping: As you sip your tea, reflect on your thoughts and feelings.

Write: Journal about your experiences, emotions, or any insights that arise during your tea time.

7. Natural Antibiotics: Combating Illnesses the Herbal Way

Chapter 31: The Crisis of Antibiotic Resistance

Antibiotics have been a cornerstone of modern medicine, saving countless lives by treating bacterial infections. However, their overuse and misuse have led to a growing crisis of antibiotic resistance, threatening our ability to combat infectious diseases effectively. In this chapter, we will delve into the complex issue of antibiotic resistance, its causes, consequences, and potential solutions.

Understanding Antibiotics

Antibiotics are drugs designed to kill or inhibit the growth of bacteria. They have been invaluable in treating bacterial infections such as pneumonia, urinary tract infections, and skin infections. However, antibiotics are powerless against viral infections like the common cold or flu.

The Rise of Antibiotic Resistance

Antibiotic resistance occurs when bacteria evolve to withstand the effects of antibiotics. This resistance can develop through various mechanisms, including:

Natural Selection: Bacteria with genetic mutations that make them resistant survive antibiotic treatment, passing on these traits to their descendants.

Overuse and Misuse: The excessive use of antibiotics, often when they are not needed or taken incorrectly (e.g., not completing a full course), accelerates the development of resistance.

Antibiotic Use in Agriculture: The use of antibiotics in agriculture for promoting animal growth and preventing disease in crowded conditions contributes to resistance.

Global Spread: Resistant bacteria can travel across borders, making antibiotic resistance a global issue.

Consequences of Antibiotic Resistance

Antibiotic resistance poses severe consequences for both individuals and society:

Limited Treatment Options: As bacteria become resistant to multiple antibiotics, infections become harder to treat, leading to longer hospital stays and increased mortality rates.

Increased Healthcare Costs: Treating resistant infections often requires more extended hospital stays, expensive medications, and additional medical procedures, leading to increased healthcare costs.

Surgery and Cancer Treatment: Routine surgeries and cancer treatments that rely on antibiotics to prevent infections become riskier when antibiotics are less effective.

Public Health Threat: Resistant bacteria can spread within communities and healthcare settings, posing a public health threat.

Addressing Antibiotic Resistance

Combatting antibiotic resistance is a complex and ongoing challenge. Several strategies are being employed:

Antibiotic Stewardship: Healthcare providers are encouraged to prescribe antibiotics only when necessary and to choose the most targeted and narrow-spectrum antibiotics.

Research and Development: Scientists are actively searching for new antibiotics and alternative treatments.

Vaccination: Preventing infections through vaccination reduces the need for antibiotics.

Public Awareness: Educating the public about the responsible use of antibiotics helps reduce demand and misuse.

Global Cooperation: International collaboration is crucial to monitoring and addressing antibiotic resistance on a global scale.

Agricultural Regulation: Reducing the use of antibiotics in agriculture and promoting responsible farming practices can help slow the development of resistance.

Personal Responsibility

Individuals can play a role in addressing antibiotic resistance:

Follow Medical Advice: Take antibiotics as prescribed, completing the full course even if you feel better.

Don't Demand Antibiotics: Trust your healthcare provider's judgment. Antibiotics are not always the answer for infections.

Practice Good Hygiene: Proper handwashing and hygiene can help prevent infections in the first place.

The Future of Antibiotics

The development of new antibiotics is essential, but it's a complex and costly process. Researchers are exploring novel approaches, including:

Phage Therapy: Using bacteriophages, viruses that infect bacteria, to treat bacterial infections.

Combination Therapy: Using multiple antibiotics or combining antibiotics with other treatments to enhance their effectiveness.

Antibacterial Peptides: Investigating naturally occurring peptides with antibacterial properties.

Chapter 32: Potent Herbal Antibiotics and Their Uses

As antibiotic resistance becomes a growing concern, there is renewed interest in herbal antibiotics — natural remedies derived from plants that have demonstrated antibacterial properties. In this chapter, we will explore several potent herbal antibiotics and their uses as alternative treatments for bacterial infections.

Garlic (Allium sativum)

Antibacterial Properties: Garlic contains allicin, a compound with strong antibacterial properties. It can combat a wide range of bacteria, including antibiotic-resistant strains.

Uses: Garlic can be consumed raw, cooked, or as a supplement. It is effective against various infections, including respiratory, digestive, and skin infections.

Echinacea (Echinacea purpurea)

Antibacterial Properties: Echinacea boosts the immune system and has antimicrobial properties that can help the body fight off infections.

Uses: Echinacea is commonly used to prevent and treat respiratory infections like colds and flu. It can also aid in wound healing.

Goldenseal (Hydrastis canadensis)

Antibacterial Properties: Goldenseal contains berberine, a potent compound with antibacterial properties. It can combat a wide range of bacteria.

Uses: Goldenseal is used for various infections, including urinary tract infections, respiratory infections, and digestive issues. It can be taken as a tincture, capsule, or in tea form.

Manuka Honey

Antibacterial Properties: Manuka honey, produced in New Zealand, has strong antibacterial properties due to its high methylglyoxal (MGO) content.

Uses: Manuka honey is applied topically to wounds and burns to prevent infection and promote healing. It can also be consumed to soothe sore throats and support overall immune health.

Thyme (Thymus vulgaris)

Antibacterial Properties: Thyme contains thymol, a compound with potent antibacterial properties effective against various bacteria.

Uses: Thyme is used in herbal teas and as a culinary herb. It can be effective in treating respiratory infections and sore throats.

Oregano (Origanum vulgare)

Antibacterial Properties: Oregano contains carvacrol and thymol, both of which have strong antibacterial properties.

Uses: Oregano oil is used to combat bacterial infections, particularly those affecting the digestive system. It can also be used as a natural food preservative.

Clove (Syzygium aromaticum)

Antibacterial Properties: Cloves contain eugenol, a compound with powerful antibacterial properties effective against various strains.

Uses: Cloves can be used in dental care to relieve toothaches and combat oral infections. Clove oil can be diluted and applied topically for skin infections.

Cinnamon (Cinnamomum verum)

Antibacterial Properties: Cinnamon contains cinnamaldehyde, a compound with antibacterial properties that can inhibit the growth of bacteria.

Uses: Cinnamon can be used in cooking, added to teas, or taken as a supplement. It may help combat digestive infections.

Ginger (Zingiber officinale)

Antibacterial Properties: Ginger has antimicrobial properties and can inhibit the growth of various bacteria.

Uses: Ginger is often used to alleviate digestive issues and nausea. It can be consumed in teas, as a spice in cooking, or as a supplement.

Cranberry (Vaccinium macrocarpon)

Antibacterial Properties: Cranberries contain proanthocyanidins that can prevent bacteria, particularly E. coli, from adhering to the urinary tract lining.

Uses: Cranberry juice or supplements are commonly used to prevent and manage urinary tract infections (UTIs).

Chapter 33: Dosage, Duration, and Safety Concerns

When using herbal antibiotics or any herbal remedies, it's crucial to understand the proper dosage, duration of use, and safety considerations. Here, we will explore these aspects to ensure that herbal treatments are used effectively and safely.

Dosage

Determining the correct dosage of herbal antibiotics is essential to achieve the desired therapeutic effects while minimizing the risk of adverse reactions. Dosage can vary depending on factors such as the herb used, the form (capsules, tinctures, teas, etc.), and the individual's age and health status. Here are some guidelines:

Follow Recommendations: Always follow the recommended dosage provided on the product label or by a qualified herbalist or healthcare provider.

Start Low: It's often advisable to start with the lowest recommended dose and gradually increase it as needed. This approach allows you to assess how your body responds.

Consult an Expert: If you're unsure about the appropriate dosage, consult with a qualified herbalist or healthcare practitioner who can provide personalized guidance.

Consider Form: The form of the herbal remedy matters. For example, tinctures are more concentrated than teas, so the dosage may differ.

Duration of Use

The duration for which you can safely use herbal antibiotics depends on the specific herb, the condition being treated, and the individual. Here are some general considerations:

Short-Term Use: Many herbal antibiotics are used for acute conditions, such as respiratory infections. In these cases, treatment is usually short-term, lasting a few days to a couple of weeks.

Chronic Conditions: For chronic conditions or recurrent infections, herbal antibiotics may be used for a more extended period, but it's essential to monitor their effects and consult with a healthcare provider regularly.

Intermittent Use: Some individuals may use herbal antibiotics intermittently, such as during cold and flu seasons or when traveling to regions with higher infection risks.

Consult a Professional: If you plan to use herbal antibiotics for an extended period, it's crucial to consult a healthcare provider or herbalist to ensure safety and effectiveness.

Safety Concerns

While herbal antibiotics offer many benefits, they are not without potential risks and safety considerations:

Allergies: Some individuals may be allergic to specific herbs. If you experience allergic reactions such as itching, rash, or swelling, discontinue use immediately.

Interactions: Herbal antibiotics can interact with medications or other herbs you may be taking. Always inform your healthcare provider of all the remedies you use to prevent adverse interactions.

Pregnancy and Nursing: Pregnant or nursing individuals should exercise caution when using herbal antibiotics. Some herbs may not be safe during these periods, so it's essential to consult with a healthcare provider.

Children and the Elderly: Dosages for children and the elderly may need adjustment. Consult with a healthcare provider or pediatrician for appropriate guidance.

Quality and Purity: Ensure you source high-quality, pure herbal products from reputable suppliers to minimize the risk of contaminants or adulterants.

Monitoring: Regularly monitor your health while using herbal antibiotics. If your condition worsens or persists, seek medical advice promptly.

Herb-Drug Interactions: Be aware of potential interactions between herbal antibiotics and prescription medications. Always inform your healthcare provider about all remedies you are using.

Self-Diagnosis: Avoid self-diagnosing serious infections. If you suspect a severe bacterial infection, seek medical attention promptly.

Chapter 34: Combining Herbs for Synergistic Effects

When it comes to herbal medicine, the combination of different herbs can often produce synergistic effects, where the combined action is greater than the sum of individual actions. This chapter explores the art and science of combining herbs to achieve enhanced therapeutic outcomes.

Understanding Synergy in Herbal Combinations

Synergy in herbal combinations occurs when the properties of two or more herbs complement each other, resulting in a more potent or balanced effect. This can involve various mechanisms, including:

Potentiation: One herb may enhance the absorption or effectiveness of another.

Complementary Actions: Herbs with different actions may work together to address multiple aspects of a health issue.

Reduced Side Effects: Combining herbs can sometimes mitigate potential side effects of individual herbs.

Balancing Properties: Synergistic combinations can balance the overall effect, making it more suitable for a specific condition or individual.

Examples of Herbal Combinations for Synergistic Effects

a. Immune Support Blend

Ingredients: Echinacea, astragalus, elderberry, and ginger.

Synergy: Echinacea stimulates the immune system, astragalus enhances immune function, elderberry provides antioxidants, and ginger offers anti-inflammatory properties. Together, they create a robust immune-supporting blend.

b. Digestive Health Blend

Ingredients: Peppermint, fennel, chamomile, and ginger.

Synergy: Peppermint soothes digestive discomfort, fennel aids digestion, chamomile calms the stomach, and ginger reduces nausea. This combination addresses various digestive issues effectively.

c. Relaxation and Sleep Aid Blend

Ingredients: Valerian root, passionflower, lemon balm, and lavender.

Synergy: Valerian induces sleep, passionflower has calming properties, lemon balm reduces stress, and lavender promotes relaxation. This blend offers comprehensive support for restful sleep.

d. Anti-Inflammatory Blend

Ingredients: Turmeric, black pepper, boswellia, and ginger.

Synergy: Turmeric reduces inflammation, black pepper enhances turmeric absorption, boswellia offers anti-inflammatory effects, and ginger adds additional anti-inflammatory properties. Together, they create a powerful anti-inflammatory blend.

Tips for Creating Herbal Combinations

a. Research and Knowledge

Understand Herb Properties: Familiarize yourself with the properties and actions of individual herbs before combining them. This knowledge helps you select complementary herbs.

Consult References: Refer to reputable herbal references, books, and resources for guidance on herbal combinations for specific conditions.

b. Start Simple

Begin with Single Herbs: When you're new to herbal combinations, start by using single herbs to address specific issues. This helps you understand each herb's effects.

Gradually Combine: As you gain experience, experiment with combining two or three herbs to address a particular health concern.

c. Seek Professional Guidance

Consult Herbalists or Healthcare Providers: If you're dealing with complex health issues or chronic conditions, consult with a qualified herbalist or healthcare provider for personalized guidance.

d. Keep Notes

Document Your Experiences: Keep a journal of the herbal combinations you try, including dosages, effects, and any side effects. This helps you refine your approach over time.

e. Be Patient

Give Time for Effects: Herbal remedies may take time to show their full effects. Be patient and consistent in your usage.

Safety and Caution

Consider Allergies: Be aware of allergies to specific herbs or their components when combining them.

Drug Interactions: Check for potential interactions with medications if you are taking any.

Pregnancy and Special Populations: Exercise caution when using herbal combinations during pregnancy, breastfeeding, or with children. Consult with a healthcare provider.

Chapter 35: Boosting Gut Health Post-Antibiotics

Antibiotics are essential for treating bacterial infections, but they can have unintended consequences on gut health. This chapter explores strategies for restoring and promoting gut health after a course of antibiotics, emphasizing the importance of a balanced and diverse gut microbiome.

Understanding the Impact of Antibiotics on Gut Health

Antibiotics are designed to target and kill harmful bacteria causing infections. However, they can also affect beneficial bacteria in the gut, disrupting the delicate balance of the microbiome. This disruption can lead to various gastrointestinal issues, including diarrhea, constipation, and susceptibility to new infections.

Probiotics: Replenishing Beneficial Bacteria

a. Probiotic Supplements: Probiotics are live beneficial bacteria that can help restore the gut microbiome. After antibiotics, taking a high-quality probiotic supplement can be beneficial. Look for products that contain a variety of bacterial strains, including Lactobacillus and Bifidobacterium species.

b. Fermented Foods: Incorporating fermented foods into your diet, such as yogurt, kefir, sauerkraut, kimchi, and kombucha, provides natural sources of probiotics. These foods can help replenish beneficial bacteria in the gut.

Prebiotics: Nourishing Your Microbiome

Prebiotics are non-digestible fibers that serve as food for beneficial bacteria in the gut. Including prebiotic-rich foods in your diet can help support the growth of these beneficial bacteria. Examples of prebiotic foods include garlic, onions, leeks, asparagus, and bananas.

Dietary Fiber: Promoting Gut Health

A diet rich in dietary fiber is essential for maintaining a healthy gut. Fiber supports regular bowel movements and provides nourishment for beneficial bacteria. Whole grains, legumes, fruits, and vegetables are excellent sources of dietary fiber.

Stay Hydrated

Adequate hydration is crucial for gut health. Water helps move food and waste through the digestive system, preventing issues like constipation. Aim to drink plenty of water throughout the day.

Avoid Excessive Sugar and Processed Foods

High sugar and processed food diets can negatively impact gut health. These foods can encourage the growth of harmful bacteria while reducing the abundance of beneficial ones. Reducing sugar intake and focusing on whole, unprocessed foods is beneficial.

Limit Antibiotic Use When Possible

Whenever feasible, avoid unnecessary antibiotic use. Antibiotics should only be taken when prescribed by a healthcare provider for a bacterial infection. Overuse or misuse of antibiotics can lead to more significant disruptions in gut health.

Incorporate Herbs and Spices

Certain herbs and spices, such as ginger, turmeric, and garlic, have natural anti-inflammatory and antimicrobial properties. Including these ingredients in your cooking can support gut health and overall well-being.

Manage Stress

Stress can affect gut health, as the gut-brain connection is well-established. Practicing stress-reduction techniques like meditation, deep breathing, and yoga can help maintain a balanced gut microbiome.

Consult a Healthcare Provider

If you experience severe gastrointestinal issues or persistent symptoms after taking antibiotics, consult a healthcare provider. They can assess your condition and provide guidance on further interventions or treatments.

8. Tinctures and Their Potency: A Deep Dive into Herbal Concentrates

Chapter 36: Tincture Basics: Alcohol vs. Glycerin-based

Tinctures are concentrated herbal extracts used for various medicinal and therapeutic purposes. They are made by macerating herbs in a liquid solvent. Two common types of solvents used for making tinctures are alcohol and glycerin. In this chapter, we will explore the differences between alcohol-based and glycerin-based tinctures, their advantages, disadvantages, and best practices for making and using them.

Alcohol-Based Tinctures

Alcohol-based tinctures use ethanol as the primary solvent. Here are some key considerations:

1. Extraction Efficiency: Alcohol is highly efficient at extracting a wide range of plant compounds, including alcohol-soluble constituents and some water-soluble ones. This makes it a versatile choice for tincture making.

2. Shelf Life: Alcohol-based tinctures typically have a longer shelf life than glycerin-based ones. The alcohol acts as a preservative, inhibiting the growth of microorganisms that can spoil the tincture.

3. Rapid Absorption: Alcohol helps facilitate the rapid absorption of herbal constituents into the bloodstream, making alcohol-based tinctures a popular choice when quick effects are desired.

4. Dosage Precision: Alcohol tinctures allow for precise dosage control due to their consistent concentration.

5. Drawbacks: Alcohol-based tinctures may not be suitable for individuals with alcohol sensitivities, including children, recovering alcoholics, or those who need to avoid alcohol for medical or personal reasons. The high alcohol content can also evaporate quickly if not stored properly.

Glycerin-Based Tinctures

Glycerin-based tinctures use glycerin as the solvent. Here are some key considerations:

1. Alcohol-Free: Glycerin-based tinctures are alcohol-free, making them a suitable option for those who cannot or prefer not to consume alcohol. They are safe for children and individuals with alcohol sensitivities.

2. Sweet Flavor: Glycerin has a naturally sweet taste, making glycerin-based tinctures more palatable, especially for children.

3. Limited Extraction: Glycerin is less efficient at extracting certain plant compounds, particularly those that are alcohol-soluble. This can result in a tincture with a milder or less comprehensive profile of herbal constituents.

4. Shorter Shelf Life: Glycerin-based tinctures generally have a shorter shelf life compared to alcohol-based ones. They may be more prone to microbial growth and spoilage over time.

5. Slower Absorption: Glycerin-based tinctures are absorbed more slowly by the body compared to alcohol-based tinctures, which may delay the onset of therapeutic effects.

Choosing Between Alcohol and Glycerin-Based Tinctures

The choice between alcohol and glycerin-based tinctures depends on individual preferences, needs, and sensitivities. Here are some considerations:

Alcohol Sensitivity: If you have alcohol sensitivities or need to avoid alcohol for any reason, glycerin-based tinctures are a suitable alternative.

Speed of Absorption: If you require rapid absorption and quick therapeutic effects, alcohol-based tinctures may be preferred.

Palatability: Glycerin-based tinctures may be more palatable, especially for children or individuals who find the taste of alcohol unpleasant.

Shelf Life: Consider the intended duration of use and storage conditions. If you plan to use the tincture quickly and can store it in a cool, dark place, glycerin-based tinctures may be sufficient.

Herb Selection: Some herbs may lend themselves better to one type of tincture over the other based on their solubility characteristics.

Chapter 37: Methods of Making Effective Tinctures

Tinctures are concentrated herbal extracts that can be made using various methods. The effectiveness of a tincture depends on the quality of the ingredients and the extraction process. In this chapter, we will explore the methods of making effective tinctures and the key factors to consider.

Selecting Quality Herbs

The quality of the herbs used is fundamental to the effectiveness of a tincture. Here are some considerations:

Choose Fresh or Dried Herbs: Fresh herbs are ideal when available, but dried herbs are more convenient and have a longer shelf life.

Source: Select high-quality herbs from reputable suppliers to ensure purity and potency.

Organic: Whenever possible, choose organic herbs to avoid exposure to pesticides and herbicides.

Choosing the Right Solvent

The choice of solvent, whether alcohol or glycerin, depends on your preferences and the herb being used. Consider the properties of the solvent and the herb to make an informed decision.

Ratio of Herb to Solvent

The ratio of herb to solvent determines the concentration of the tincture. Generally, a common ratio is 1:5, meaning one part of herb to five parts of solvent. However, this ratio can vary based on the herb's strength and the desired potency.

Maceration Time

Maceration is the process of allowing the herbs to steep in the solvent. The duration of maceration can range from a few days to several weeks, depending on the herb and the desired strength of the tincture. Be sure to follow specific guidelines for the herb you are using.

Temperature and Light

Store the tincture during maceration in a cool, dark place. Exposure to heat and light can degrade the quality of the tincture. Amber glass bottles can help protect the tincture from light.

Agitation

Some herbalists recommend gently shaking or stirring the tincture daily during the maceration process to enhance extraction.

Straining and Pressing

After the maceration period, strain the tincture to remove the plant material. You can use a fine mesh strainer or cheesecloth. For maximum extraction, press the remaining herbs to extract any trapped liquid.

Storage

Store the tincture in amber glass bottles with tight-fitting lids to protect it from light and air. Label the bottles with the herb, solvent used, date of preparation, and any specific instructions or warnings.

Dosage and Dilution

The effectiveness of a tincture also depends on proper dosage and dilution. Be sure to follow recommended dosage guidelines for the specific tincture and consult with a healthcare provider if necessary.

Testing and Quality Control

Consider having your tinctures tested for potency and purity by a reputable laboratory, especially if you plan to sell them or use them for serious health conditions.

Legal and Safety Considerations

Be aware of the legal and safety considerations when making tinctures. Some herbs may have restrictions or safety concerns, so it's essential to research and follow guidelines.

Chapter 38: Dosage, Duration, and Best Practices

Using herbal remedies effectively requires an understanding of proper dosage, duration of use, and best practices to ensure safety and efficacy. This chapter explores these critical aspects of herbal medicine.

Dosage

Determining the correct dosage of herbal remedies is essential for achieving the desired therapeutic effects while minimizing the risk of adverse reactions. Dosage can vary depending on factors such as the herb used, the form (tinctures, teas, capsules, etc.), and individual factors like age and health status. Here are some guidelines:

Follow Recommendations: Always follow the recommended dosage provided on the product label or by a qualified herbalist or healthcare provider.

Start Low: It's often advisable to start with the lowest recommended dose and gradually increase it as needed. This approach allows you to assess how your body responds.

Consult an Expert: If you're unsure about the appropriate dosage, consult with a qualified herbalist or healthcare practitioner who can provide personalized guidance.

Consider Form: The form of the herbal remedy matters. For example, tinctures are more concentrated than teas, so the dosage may differ.

Duration of Use

The duration for which you can safely use herbal remedies depends on the specific herb, the condition being treated, and the individual. Here are some general considerations:

Short-Term Use: Many herbal remedies are used for acute conditions, such as colds or digestive issues. In these cases, treatment is usually short-term, lasting a few days to a couple of weeks.

Chronic Conditions: For chronic conditions or ongoing health support, herbal remedies may be used for a more extended period, but it's essential to monitor their effects and consult with a healthcare provider regularly.

Intermittent Use: Some individuals may use herbal remedies intermittently, such as during specific seasons or when experiencing particular symptoms.

Consult a Professional: If you plan to use herbal remedies for an extended period or have a complex health issue, it's crucial to consult a healthcare provider or herbalist to ensure safety and effectiveness.

Quality and Sourcing

The quality of the herbs used in herbal remedies is vital for their efficacy. Here are some considerations:

Reputable Suppliers: Source herbs from reputable suppliers who adhere to quality standards and provide detailed information about the source and processing of their products.

Organic and Sustainable: Whenever possible, choose organic herbs to minimize exposure to pesticides and herbicides. Additionally, consider herbs sourced through sustainable and ethical practices.

Purity: Ensure that the herbs you use are free from contaminants or adulterants. High-quality herbs contribute to the overall effectiveness of the remedy.

Monitoring and Adjusting

When using herbal remedies, it's crucial to monitor your health and adjust the treatment as needed. Here are some tips:

Regular Check-Ins: Pay attention to how your body responds to the herbal remedy. If you experience unexpected side effects or if your condition worsens, seek medical advice promptly.

Adjust Dosage: If you don't experience the desired effects, consider adjusting the dosage or trying a different herbal remedy under the guidance of a qualified herbalist or healthcare provider.

Be Patient: Herbal remedies may take time to show their full effects. Be patient and consistent in your usage.

Safety and Contraindications

It's essential to be aware of potential safety concerns and contraindications when using herbal remedies:

Allergies: Some individuals may be allergic to specific herbs. If you experience allergic reactions such as itching, rash, or swelling, discontinue use immediately.

Interactions: Herbal remedies can interact with medications or other herbs you may be taking. Always inform your healthcare provider of all the remedies you use to prevent adverse interactions.

Special Populations: Pregnant or nursing individuals, children, and the elderly may require adjusted dosages or specific precautions. Consult with a healthcare provider or pediatrician for appropriate guidance.

Quality and Purity: Ensure you source high-quality, pure herbal products from reputable suppliers to minimize the risk of contaminants or adulterants.

Herb-Drug Interactions

Be aware of potential interactions between herbal remedies and prescription medications. Always inform your healthcare provider about all remedies you are using to avoid any adverse effects or interactions.

Chapter 39: Special Tinctures: Vinegars, Honeys, and Wines

In addition to traditional alcohol and glycerin-based tinctures, herbalists have long utilized other mediums like vinegars, honeys, and wines to extract and preserve the medicinal properties of herbs. These special tinctures offer unique flavors and therapeutic benefits.

Herbal Vinegars

Herbal vinegars involve macerating herbs in vinegar, typically apple cider vinegar. They are valued for their tangy taste and versatility in culinary and medicinal applications.

Preparation: To make an herbal vinegar, fill a glass jar with fresh or dried herbs, leaving some space at the top. Pour room-temperature vinegar over the herbs until they are fully covered. Seal the jar and store it in a cool, dark place for several weeks, shaking it daily. After the maceration period, strain the vinegar and transfer it to a clean bottle.

Uses:

Culinary: Herbal vinegars can be used as salad dressings, marinades, or flavor enhancers in cooking.

Medicinal: Herbal vinegars can be used medicinally, often diluted in water, for various health benefits such as digestive support or immune boosting.

Herbal Honeys

Herbal honeys involve infusing honey with herbs to create a sweet and medicinally potent concoction.

Preparation: To make herbal honey, place fresh or dried herbs in a clean glass jar. Pour honey over the herbs, ensuring they are fully submerged. Seal the jar and allow it to sit in a warm, sunny location for several weeks. Stir or shake it occasionally. Afterward, strain the honey to remove the herbs.

Uses:

Cough and Cold Relief: Herbal honeys with herbs like thyme or sage can be soothing for sore throats and coughs.

Immune Support: Some herbal honeys, such as elderberry honey, can provide immune-boosting benefits.

Flavor Enhancer: Herbal honeys can be added to tea, yogurt, or toast for added flavor and health benefits.

Herbal Wines

Herbal wines involve steeping herbs in wine, usually a dry white or red wine. They are appreciated for their rich flavors and therapeutic qualities.

Preparation: To make herbal wine, place your chosen herbs in a glass jar and cover them with wine. Seal the jar and let it sit in a cool, dark place for a few weeks, shaking it occasionally. After the maceration period, strain the wine to remove the herbs.

Uses:

Digestive Aid: Herbal wines can serve as digestive tonics, taken in small quantities before or after meals to support digestion.

Relaxation: Certain herbal wines, like lavender or chamomile-infused wine, can promote relaxation and better sleep.

Culinary: Herbal wines can also be used in cooking, adding unique flavors to dishes.

Safety Considerations:

Alcohol Content: Herbal wines contain alcohol, so they should be consumed in moderation, especially if driving or operating machinery.

Allergies: Be cautious if you have allergies to specific herbs or components in the herbal preparations.

Pregnancy and Special Populations: Pregnant individuals and those with specific health conditions should consult with a healthcare provider before using herbal wines or other alcoholic herbal preparations.

Chapter 40: Storing and Labeling: Keeping Tinctures Organized

Proper storage and labeling are crucial aspects of herbal medicine. Ensuring that your tinctures are stored correctly and labeled accurately not only maintains their potency but also prevents mix-ups and enhances safety.

Storing Tinctures

Storing tinctures correctly helps preserve their quality and potency over time. Here's how to do it:

Dark Glass Bottles: Tinctures should be stored in dark glass bottles, typically amber or cobalt blue, to protect them from light, which can degrade their quality.

Cool, Dark Place: Store tinctures in a cool, dark place, away from direct sunlight and temperature fluctuations. A cupboard or pantry is an ideal location.

Tight Seals: Ensure that the bottle caps or dropper lids are tightly sealed to prevent air from entering, which can lead to spoilage or evaporation.

Label Placement: Store tinctures upright to prevent leakage and label smudging.

Avoiding Contamination: Use clean droppers or pipettes when dispensing tinctures to avoid contamination.

Labeling Tinctures

Clear and accurate labeling is essential for safety and organization. Here's how to label tinctures effectively:

Name of Herb: Clearly state the name of the herb used in the tincture. Include both the common and scientific names if possible.

Type of Solvent: Indicate whether the tincture is alcohol-based, glycerin-based, vinegar-based, etc.

Date of Preparation: Include the date when the tincture was made. This helps track its freshness and potency.

Dosage Instructions: Specify the recommended dosage for adults and any special instructions. If the tincture is intended for children or specific populations, include separate dosing instructions.

Safety Information: Note any safety precautions or contraindications. For example, if the herb is not suitable for pregnant individuals, mention it.

Batch Number: Assign a unique batch number to each tincture you prepare. This can be helpful for quality control and tracking.

Alcohol Content: For alcohol-based tinctures, it's helpful to include the percentage of alcohol, especially if it's higher than the standard 40-60%.

Extraction Time: Mention the duration for which the herbs were macerated in the solvent.

Storage Instructions: Include guidelines for storing the tincture correctly.

Additional Notes: You can add any other relevant information, such as the source of the herbs or the intended use.

Organizing Tinctures

Organizing your tinctures efficiently can save time and prevent mix-ups. Consider these tips:

Shelving: Use dedicated shelves or cabinets for your tincture collection. Arrange them in alphabetical order or by category for easy access.

Color Coding: Assign different colors to labels or caps to quickly identify tinctures with specific properties or purposes (e.g., blue for calming herbs, red for energizing herbs).

Inventory List: Maintain an inventory list or spreadsheet to keep track of the tinctures you have, their quantities, and expiration dates.

Rotation: Use the oldest tinctures first to ensure freshness and potency. Label bottles with their preparation date to help with rotation.

9. Safety First: Side Effects and Interactions of Herbal Remedies

Chapter 41: Recognizing Herbal Allergies and Sensitivities

While herbal remedies are generally considered safe, it's essential to be aware that individuals can have allergies or sensitivities to specific herbs. Recognizing these allergies and sensitivities is crucial for safe and effective herbal medicine practice.

Common Herbal Allergens

Several herbs are more commonly associated with allergic reactions. Some of these include:

Echinacea: While often used to boost the immune system, echinacea can trigger allergic reactions in some individuals, especially those with allergies to plants in the Asteraceae family.

Chamomile: Chamomile is generally gentle, but it can cause allergic reactions, particularly in individuals with ragweed allergies.

St. John's Wort: This herb may cause skin sensitivity to sunlight in some individuals, resulting in skin rashes or burns when exposed to the sun.

Aloe Vera: While usually used topically, some people may experience skin reactions to aloe vera.

Ginkgo Biloba: Ginkgo supplements have been associated with allergic skin reactions in some cases.

Lavender: Although lavender is well-tolerated by most, it can cause skin irritation or allergies in sensitive individuals.

Recognizing Allergic Reactions

Allergic reactions to herbs can manifest in various ways:

Skin Reactions: This includes itching, redness, hives, or rashes upon contact with or use of the herb.

Respiratory Symptoms: Allergies can lead to symptoms like sneezing, nasal congestion, coughing, or wheezing.

Gastrointestinal Distress: Some individuals may experience nausea, vomiting, diarrhea, or abdominal pain due to herbal allergies.

Anaphylaxis: In severe cases, an allergic reaction can be life-threatening, causing difficulty breathing, swelling of the face or throat, rapid heartbeat, and a drop in blood pressure. This is a medical emergency.

Sensitivities vs. Allergies

It's important to distinguish between sensitivities and allergies:

Sensitivities: Sensitivities may cause discomfort or mild symptoms but are not as severe as allergies. They can develop over time with repeated exposure.

Allergies: Allergic reactions are typically more immediate and severe. They can occur even with minimal exposure to the allergen and may worsen with each subsequent exposure.

Cross-Reactivity

Cross-reactivity can occur when an individual is allergic to one substance and experiences a similar allergic reaction when exposed to a related substance. For example, if someone is allergic to ragweed, they may also react to chamomile, which belongs to the same plant family.

Testing for Allergies

If you suspect an allergy to a specific herb or are at risk due to known allergies, consider allergy testing. Skin prick tests and blood tests (such as specific IgE tests) can help identify allergies to herbs and other substances.

Precautions and Avoidance

If you have known allergies or sensitivities to specific herbs, it's crucial to:

Read Labels: Carefully read product labels and ingredient lists to avoid products containing the allergen.

Consult Professionals: Consult with a qualified herbalist or healthcare provider who can recommend alternative herbs or therapies that do not trigger allergies.

Patch Testing: Perform a patch test before using herbs topically, especially if you have sensitive skin.

Start Slowly: When trying a new herbal remedy, start with a small dose to gauge your body's response.

Monitor for Reactions: Pay close attention to your body's reactions when using herbs and seek medical attention if you experience allergic symptoms.

Chapter 42: Potential Interactions with Prescription Drugs

The use of herbal remedies alongside prescription drugs is a topic of increasing importance as people seek complementary or alternative approaches to healthcare. While herbs can offer various health benefits, it's essential to be aware of potential interactions between herbs and prescription medications to ensure safety and effectiveness.

Understanding Drug-Herb Interactions

Drug-herb interactions occur when the compounds in herbs affect the absorption, metabolism, or elimination of prescription medications in the body. These interactions can result in changes in drug levels, potentially reducing their efficacy or increasing the risk of side effects.

Types of Drug-Herb Interactions

There are several types of drug-herb interactions to be aware of:

Pharmacokinetic Interactions: These interactions affect how drugs are absorbed, metabolized, distributed, or excreted. For example, an herb may inhibit or induce liver enzymes responsible for drug metabolism, altering drug levels in the body.

Pharmacodynamic Interactions: These interactions occur when herbs and drugs with similar or opposing effects on the body are used together, potentially intensifying or diminishing therapeutic effects. For example, combining a blood-thinning herb with an anticoagulant medication can increase the risk of bleeding.

Pharmacokinetic-Pharmacodynamic Interactions: These interactions involve a combination of effects on drug metabolism and drug action. They can be complex and challenging to predict.

Common Herb-Drug Interactions

Certain herbs are more likely to interact with specific classes of drugs:

Blood-Thinning Herbs: Herbs like garlic, ginger, ginkgo biloba, and turmeric have mild blood-thinning properties. When combined with anticoagulant medications (e.g., warfarin), they can increase the risk of bleeding.

St. John's Wort: This herb is known to induce liver enzymes, potentially reducing the effectiveness of various medications, including antidepressants, oral contraceptives, and antiretroviral drugs used in HIV treatment.

Grapefruit: While not an herb, grapefruit and its juice can interact with a wide range of medications by inhibiting certain enzymes responsible for drug metabolism, leading to higher drug concentrations in the blood.

Licorice: Licorice root can affect potassium levels in the body, which can be problematic when combined with medications that also affect potassium levels, such as certain blood pressure medications.

Individual Variability

Interactions between herbs and drugs can vary from person to person. Factors such as genetics, dosage, and the specific combination of herbs and drugs play a role in determining the extent of the interaction.

Precautions and Consultation

To minimize the risk of herb-drug interactions:

Consult a Healthcare Provider: Before starting any herbal remedy, consult with a qualified healthcare provider who can assess your specific health needs and potential interactions.

Full Disclosure: Provide your healthcare provider with a comprehensive list of all medications, supplements, and herbs you are using.

Herbalist Consultation: Seek guidance from a qualified herbalist who is knowledgeable about potential interactions and can recommend appropriate herbs.

Start Slowly: If you decide to use herbs alongside medications, start with a low dose of the herb to monitor your body's response.

Regular Monitoring: If using herbs and drugs together, your healthcare provider may need to monitor your health more closely to ensure safety and effectiveness.

Chapter 43: Age-Specific Considerations: Children and Elderly

Herbal medicine is a versatile approach to healthcare, but it's important to recognize that different age groups, such as children and the elderly, have unique considerations when it comes to using herbs for health and wellness.

Children and Herbal Medicine

Children's bodies are still developing, and they may react differently to herbs compared to adults. Here are some key considerations when using herbs for children:

Dosing: Children typically require lower doses of herbs compared to adults. Dosages should be based on the child's age, weight, and the specific herb being used. Pediatric herbalists can provide guidance on appropriate dosing.

Safety: Some herbs may not be safe for children. It's essential to choose herbs that are well-tolerated and appropriate for the child's age and health condition.

Formulation: Herbal remedies for children are often prepared in forms that are easier for them to take, such as glycerites, syrups, or teas sweetened with honey.

Consultation: Always consult with a pediatrician or qualified herbalist before giving herbs to children. They can provide guidance on suitable remedies and dosages.

Allergies and Sensitivities: Children may have allergies or sensitivities to certain herbs, so it's crucial to start with a small dose and monitor for adverse reactions.

Taste: Consider the taste of herbal remedies, as children may be more willing to take herbs that are palatable. Sweet-tasting herbs like chamomile or elderberry are often more appealing to kids.

The Elderly and Herbal Medicine

As people age, their bodies undergo changes that can affect how they respond to herbs. Here are some considerations when using herbs for the elderly:

Metabolism: Aging can lead to changes in metabolism and organ function, affecting how herbs are absorbed and processed in the body. Dosages may need to be adjusted accordingly.

Polypharmacy: The elderly often take multiple prescription medications. There is a higher risk of herb-drug interactions, so it's crucial to consult with a healthcare provider who is knowledgeable about both herbs and pharmaceuticals.

Digestive Health: Age-related changes in digestive function can affect the absorption of herbs. Tinctures and teas may be better tolerated than capsules or pills.

Cognitive Health: Some herbs, like Ginkgo biloba, are used to support cognitive function in the elderly. However, it's important to use them under the guidance of a healthcare provider, as they can interact with medications for cognitive conditions.

Bone Health: Herbs like horsetail are sometimes used to support bone health in the elderly, but their use should be supervised, especially if the person is taking medications for osteoporosis.

Kidney and Liver Function: Aging can affect kidney and liver function, which play a role in metabolizing and excreting herbs. Be cautious with herbs that have potential nephrotoxic or hepatotoxic effects.

Individualized Approach

Both for children and the elderly, an individualized approach is essential. Consider the person's overall health, specific health conditions, medications they are taking, and any allergies or sensitivities they may have.

Consultation with Healthcare Providers

Whether dealing with children or the elderly, it's advisable to consult with healthcare providers who have expertise in herbal medicine. Pediatricians can provide guidance for children, and geriatricians or integrative medicine practitioners can assist the elderly.

Chapter 44: Herbs to Avoid During Pregnancy and Lactation

Pregnancy and lactation are critical phases in a woman's life, and caution should be exercised when using herbs during these times. While some herbs can be beneficial during pregnancy and lactation, there are several that should be avoided due to potential risks. Here's a detailed explanation of herbs to avoid during these stages:

Pregnancy:

During pregnancy, the developing fetus is sensitive to substances that can cross the placental barrier. It's crucial to avoid herbs that may have adverse effects on pregnancy, including:

1. **Pennyroyal (Mentha pulegium):** Pennyroyal is a potent emmenagogue, meaning it can stimulate uterine contractions. Ingesting pennyroyal during pregnancy can lead to miscarriage and should be strictly avoided.

2. **Black and Blue Cohosh (Cimicifuga racemosa and Caulophyllum thalictroides):** These herbs are known for their potential to induce labor and should only be used under the guidance of a qualified healthcare provider during the final stages of pregnancy to assist with childbirth.

3. **Tansy (Tanacetum vulgare):** Tansy contains compounds like thujone, which can be harmful during pregnancy. It may cause uterine contractions and should be avoided.

4. **Wormwood (Artemisia absinthium):** Wormwood contains thujone and should be avoided during pregnancy due to its potential to cause uterine contractions and harm the developing fetus.

5. **Goldenseal (Hydrastis canadensis):** Goldenseal contains berberine, which may cause uterine contractions and should be avoided during pregnancy.

6. **Saw Palmetto (Serenoa repens):** Saw palmetto is sometimes used for prostate health but should be avoided during pregnancy as it may have hormonal effects.

7. **Dong Quai (Angelica sinensis):** Dong quai is known for its potential to stimulate uterine contractions and should not be used during pregnancy.

Lactation:

When breastfeeding, substances from the mother's diet and herbs can pass into breast milk and affect the nursing infant. While some herbs are considered safe during lactation, others should be used cautiously or avoided:

1. **Sage (Salvia officinalis):** Sage can reduce milk production and should be used sparingly during lactation.

2. **Peppermint (Mentha piperita):** Peppermint can also decrease milk supply and should be consumed in moderation.

3. **Parsley (Petroselinum crispum):** Parsley has mild diuretic properties and should be used in culinary amounts rather than as a concentrated supplement during breastfeeding.

4. **Oregano (Origanum vulgare):** Oregano can reduce milk supply and should be used in moderation in culinary preparations.

5. **Ginseng (Panax ginseng):** Ginseng can have stimulant effects and may affect the nursing infant's sleep patterns. It's best used cautiously or avoided.

6. **Echinacea (Echinacea spp.):** While echinacea is generally considered safe, some experts recommend using it with caution during lactation due to the potential for allergenic compounds to pass into breast milk.

7. **St. John's Wort (Hypericum perforatum):** St. John's Wort can have mood-altering effects and should be avoided during lactation due to concerns about its impact on the nursing infant's mood.

Consultation with Healthcare Providers:

If you are pregnant or breastfeeding and considering the use of herbal remedies, it's crucial to consult with healthcare providers knowledgeable about herbal medicine. They can provide guidance on safe herbs, appropriate dosages, and potential risks. Always disclose your pregnancy or lactation status when discussing herbal use with healthcare providers.

Chapter 45: Overdose Symptoms and Emergency Protocols

Using herbal remedies can provide numerous health benefits, but it's important to recognize that, like any substances, herbs can have adverse effects when consumed in excessive amounts. This chapter discusses overdose symptoms associated with herbs and outlines emergency protocols for handling herbal overdose situations.

Overdose Symptoms:

Overdose symptoms can vary widely depending on the herb, its potency, and the individual's sensitivity. Some common overdose symptoms associated with herbs include:

1. **Gastrointestinal Distress:** Overconsumption of certain herbs may lead to nausea, vomiting, diarrhea, or abdominal pain.

2. **Dizziness and Headaches:** Some herbs, especially those with psychoactive properties, may cause dizziness, headaches, or altered consciousness when taken in excess.

3. **Allergic Reactions:** Allergic reactions can manifest as skin rashes, itching, swelling, hives, or difficulty breathing.

4. **Cardiovascular Effects:** Certain herbs can affect heart rate and blood pressure, potentially leading to palpitations or chest pain.

5. **Liver or Kidney Problems:** Overdosing on herbs can sometimes lead to liver or kidney damage, with symptoms like dark urine, jaundice, or abdominal discomfort.

6. **Neurological Symptoms:** In extreme cases, overdose may result in seizures, hallucinations, or other neurological symptoms.

Emergency Protocols:

If you suspect that you or someone else has overdosed on herbs, follow these emergency protocols:

1. **Call for Help:** Dial emergency services immediately if the individual experiences severe symptoms, such as difficulty breathing, seizures, or loss of consciousness.

2. **Contact Poison Control:** In non-life-threatening situations, contact your local poison control center or a healthcare provider. They can provide guidance on managing the situation and may advise on whether

to seek medical attention.

3. Gather Information: If possible, gather information about the herb consumed, the amount ingested, and the time of ingestion. This information will be valuable for healthcare professionals.

4. Do Not Induce Vomiting: Avoid inducing vomiting unless instructed to do so by a healthcare professional. Some herbs can be caustic and may cause further damage when brought back up.

5. Stay Hydrated: Encourage the individual to drink water or clear fluids to help flush the herb from their system. However, avoid excessive fluid intake, as this can be harmful.

6. Monitor Vital Signs: Keep an eye on the individual's vital signs, such as pulse, breathing rate, and blood pressure, if possible. Report any significant changes to healthcare professionals.

7. Seek Medical Evaluation: Even if symptoms appear mild, it's advisable to seek medical evaluation. Some herbs may have delayed or cumulative effects that require monitoring.

Prevention:

Preventing herbal overdose is essential for safety:

Follow Dosage Recommendations: Always adhere to recommended dosages provided by qualified herbalists or on product labels. More is not necessarily better with herbal remedies.

Keep Records: Maintain records of the herbs you are using, including dosages and administration times. This can help you track your usage and detect any potential issues.

Consult Professionals: Seek guidance from healthcare providers or herbalists experienced in herbal medicine to ensure safe and appropriate use of herbs.

Be Informed: Educate yourself about the herbs you are using, including potential side effects and interactions with medications.

Store Safely: Store herbs in a cool, dry place away from direct sunlight and out of the reach of children.

10. The Herb Directory: Detailed Profiles of Popular Healing Plants

Chapter 46: Roots: From Ginseng to Valerian

Herbal roots have a rich history in traditional medicine systems worldwide. They are valued for their diverse therapeutic properties and have been used for centuries to address various health concerns. In this chapter, we explore some notable herbal roots, including Ginseng, Echinacea, and Valerian, highlighting their uses and benefits.

Ginseng (Panax ginseng):

- Ginseng is one of the most renowned adaptogenic herbs, known for its ability to help the body adapt to stress and boost energy levels.
- It is commonly used to enhance vitality, improve cognitive function, and support the immune system.
- Ginseng may help regulate blood sugar levels, promote cardiovascular health, and enhance endurance and stamina.
- This root is often consumed as a tea or taken in the form of supplements.

Echinacea (Echinacea purpurea):

- Echinacea is a well-known immune-boosting herb, primarily used to prevent and alleviate the symptoms of the common cold and flu.
- It has anti-inflammatory and antioxidant properties that support the body's defense mechanisms.
- Echinacea root is used to make tinctures, capsules, teas, and topical preparations.
- It is best taken at the onset of illness or as a preventive measure during cold and flu season.

Valerian (Valeriana officinalis):

- Valerian root is a popular herb for promoting relaxation, reducing anxiety, and improving sleep quality.
- It is often used as a natural remedy for insomnia and other sleep disorders.
- Valerian root may help calm the nervous system, making it a valuable option for managing stress and anxiety.
- It is available in various forms, such as capsules, tinctures, and teas.

Licorice (Glycyrrhiza glabra):

- Licorice root is known for its sweet flavor and its ability to soothe coughs and sore throats.
- It has anti-inflammatory properties and may help with digestive issues, such as heartburn and gastritis.
- Licorice root is used in traditional Chinese medicine (TCM) to harmonize herbal formulas and enhance their effectiveness.
- It can be consumed as a tea or used in powdered form in herbal blends.

Dandelion (Taraxacum officinale):

- Dandelion root is used to support liver health and promote digestion.
- It is considered a natural diuretic, aiding in the elimination of excess fluids and toxins from the body.
- Dandelion root is also a source of vitamins and minerals, including potassium and vitamin C.
- It can be consumed as a tea or used in roasted form as a coffee substitute.

Burdock (Arctium lappa):

- Burdock root is valued for its detoxifying properties and its role in promoting clear and healthy skin.
- It supports the liver's natural detoxification processes and may help with skin conditions like acne.
- Burdock root can be consumed as a tea, used in culinary dishes, or taken as a supplement.

Astragalus (Astragalus membranaceus):

- Astragalus root is commonly used in traditional Chinese medicine (TCM) to strengthen the immune system and increase vitality.
- It may help reduce the frequency and severity of colds and respiratory infections.
- Astragalus root is often simmered as a soup or brewed into a tea.
- It is considered an adaptogen, helping the body adapt to stress and improve overall resilience.

These herbal roots offer a diverse range of health benefits and can be valuable additions to your natural health toolkit. However, it's important to use them mindfully and, if needed, consult with a qualified herbalist or healthcare provider to determine the most appropriate and effective way to incorporate them into your wellness routine.

Chapter 47: Leaves: From Nettle to Peppermint

Leaves of various plants have been used for their medicinal properties and culinary applications for centuries. In this chapter, we explore a selection of noteworthy herbal leaves, including Nettle, Peppermint, and Lemon Balm, highlighting their uses and benefits.

Nettle (Urtica dioica):

- Nettle leaves are rich in vitamins, minerals, and antioxidants, making them a popular choice for herbal teas and supplements.
- They are known for their ability to support allergy relief and reduce symptoms like sneezing and itching.
- Nettle leaves may help regulate blood sugar levels and contribute to overall immune system health.
- They are commonly consumed as a tea, added to soups, or used as a supplement.

Peppermint (Mentha piperita):

- Peppermint leaves are well-known for their refreshing flavor and soothing properties.
- They are often used to alleviate digestive discomfort, such as bloating, gas, and indigestion.
- Peppermint tea can help relax the muscles of the gastrointestinal tract and provide relief from irritable bowel syndrome (IBS) symptoms.
- This versatile herb can also be used to make aromatic essential oil.

Lemon Balm (Melissa officinalis):

- Lemon balm leaves have a pleasant lemony scent and are used to promote relaxation and reduce stress and anxiety.
- They have mild sedative properties and can aid in improving sleep quality.
- Lemon balm is often used in herbal blends for its calming effects.
- It can be consumed as a tea, taken as a tincture, or used in aromatherapy.

Chamomile (Matricaria chamomilla):

- Chamomile leaves, known for their apple-like aroma, are commonly used to relieve anxiety and promote relaxation.

- They are prized for their ability to soothe digestive discomfort, including indigestion and gas.
- Chamomile tea is a popular choice for calming nerves and improving sleep.
- It is also used topically in skin care products for its anti-inflammatory properties.

Raspberry Leaf (Rubus idaeus):

- Raspberry leaves are used primarily for their benefits during pregnancy and childbirth.
- They are believed to strengthen the uterine muscles and potentially reduce the duration of labor.
- Raspberry leaf tea is often recommended for pregnant individuals in their third trimester.
- It can also be consumed for general uterine health.

Holy Basil (Ocimum sanctum):

- Holy basil leaves, also known as Tulsi, are revered in Ayurvedic medicine for their adaptogenic properties.
- They are used to combat stress, support cognitive function, and boost immunity.
- Holy basil leaves are often consumed as a tea or taken in supplement form.
- They are considered a sacred herb in Hinduism and are used in rituals.

Rosemary (Rosmarinus officinalis):

- Rosemary leaves are aromatic and are commonly used as a culinary herb to flavor dishes.
- They contain antioxidants and may have anti-inflammatory properties.
- Rosemary essential oil is used in aromatherapy and for topical applications.
- The leaves can be dried and used in herbal teas or added to infused oils.

These herbal leaves offer a wide array of health benefits, from digestive relief to stress reduction. Incorporating them into your daily routine, whether through teas, culinary applications, or supplements, can enhance your overall well-being. However, it's essential to use them mindfully and, if needed, consult with a qualified herbalist or healthcare provider for personalized guidance on their use.

Chapter 48: Flowers: From Chamomile to Lavender

Flowers have long been cherished for their beauty, fragrance, and therapeutic properties. In this chapter, we explore several remarkable floral herbs, including Chamomile, Lavender, and Calendula, highlighting their diverse uses and benefits.

Chamomile (Matricaria chamomilla):

- Chamomile flowers are renowned for their calming and soothing properties, both internally and topically.
- Chamomile tea is a popular remedy for anxiety, insomnia, and digestive discomfort.
- It has anti-inflammatory and antioxidant effects, making it useful for various skin conditions when used in topical preparations.
- Chamomile essential oil is also valued in aromatherapy for relaxation.

Lavender (Lavandula angustifolia):

- Lavender flowers are celebrated for their pleasant aroma and versatile uses.
- Lavender essential oil is known for its calming and stress-relieving properties. It can be used in aromatherapy and applied topically.
- Lavender tea is consumed for relaxation and improved sleep.
- It has antimicrobial properties and can be used topically for minor burns, insect bites, and skin irritations.

Calendula (Calendula officinalis):

- Calendula flowers have anti-inflammatory and wound-healing properties, making them valuable in topical preparations.
- Calendula-infused oil is used for soothing and healing various skin conditions, such as cuts, bruises, and rashes.
- It is often included in herbal salves and creams for skin care.
- Calendula tea can be consumed for its mild anti-inflammatory effects and potential digestive benefits.

Elderflower (Sambucus nigra):

- Elderflower is revered for its immune-boosting properties and its use in combating colds and flu.
- It is often prepared as a tea, syrup, or tincture to relieve respiratory congestion and reduce fever.
- Elderflower's diaphoretic action can promote sweating, aiding the body's natural response to infections.
- The flowers are also used in culinary creations like elderflower cordial and elderflower fritters.

Hibiscus (Hibiscus sabdariffa):

- Hibiscus flowers are known for their vibrant red color and tart flavor.
- Hibiscus tea is rich in antioxidants and is consumed for its potential cardiovascular benefits, including blood pressure management.
- It has a cooling effect and is a popular choice for refreshing iced teas.
- Hibiscus flowers can also be used as a natural dye for fabrics and foods.

Rose (Rosa spp.):

- Rose petals are not only visually appealing but also offer a range of therapeutic benefits.
- Rosewater, derived from distilling rose petals, is used in skincare for its hydrating and soothing properties.
- Rose tea has a delicate floral flavor and may help relieve stress and support digestion.
- Rose essential oil is valued in aromatherapy for its emotional balancing effects.

Yarrow (Achillea millefolium):

- Yarrow flowers are known for their astringent and anti-inflammatory properties.
- Yarrow tea is traditionally used to reduce fever, promote sweating, and support overall immune health.
- It can be used topically in poultices or infused oils for wound healing.
- Yarrow's botanical name, Achillea, is derived from the legend that Achilles used the herb to treat soldiers' wounds.

These floral herbs offer a delightful blend of sensory pleasure and therapeutic value. Whether you enjoy them as teas, incorporate them into skincare routines, or explore their aromatic properties, these flowers have much to offer in terms of holistic well-being. As with any herbal use, it's advisable to use them responsibly and seek guidance from qualified herbalists or healthcare providers when necessary.

Chapter 49: Seeds and Berries: From Fennel to Goji

Seeds and berries from various plants have played essential roles in both culinary and medicinal traditions around the world. In this chapter, we explore a selection of noteworthy seeds and berries, including Fennel, Chia, and Goji berries, highlighting their diverse uses and health benefits.

Fennel Seeds (Foeniculum vulgare):

- Fennel seeds are known for their distinct licorice-like flavor and are used as a spice in cooking.
- They have digestive properties and can help alleviate gas, bloating, and indigestion.
- Fennel tea is consumed for its potential to promote lactation in breastfeeding mothers.
- These seeds are also rich in antioxidants and may have anti-inflammatory effects.

Chia Seeds (Salvia hispanica):

- Chia seeds are tiny powerhouses packed with nutrients like omega-3 fatty acids, fiber, and protein.
- They are a popular addition to smoothies, yogurt, and oatmeal, as they can help promote satiety and digestive regularity.
- Chia seeds absorb liquid and form a gel-like consistency, making them suitable for puddings and beverages.
- They offer sustained energy and can be part of a balanced diet.

Goji Berries (Lycium barbarum):

- Goji berries, also known as wolfberries, are celebrated for their high antioxidant content and potential immune-boosting properties.
- They are consumed as a snack, added to trail mixes, or used in smoothies and desserts.
- Goji berries are believed to support eye health and may help reduce the risk of age-related macular degeneration.
- They have a mildly sweet and tangy flavor, making them a versatile addition to recipes.

Flax Seeds (Linum usitatissimum):

- Flax seeds are rich in omega-3 fatty acids, fiber, and lignans, which have potential health benefits.
- Ground flax seeds are often used as a natural egg substitute in vegan baking.

- They can help lower cholesterol levels and may have a protective effect against certain cancers.
- Flax seeds can be sprinkled on cereal, added to smoothies, or used in baking recipes.

Black Sesame Seeds (Sesamum indicum):

- Black sesame seeds are a common ingredient in Asian cuisine and are used for their nutty flavor and visual appeal.
- They are a good source of calcium, iron, and healthy fats.
- Black sesame seeds are often ground into a paste to make tahini, a staple in Middle Eastern cuisine.
- In traditional Chinese medicine (TCM), they are believed to nourish the kidneys and promote hair health.

Cranberries (Vaccinium macrocarpon):

- Cranberries are well-known for their tart flavor and are often consumed in various forms, including dried, fresh, and as juice.
- They are valued for their potential to prevent urinary tract infections (UTIs) by inhibiting bacteria from adhering to the bladder lining.
- Cranberries are rich in antioxidants and vitamin C, supporting overall immune health.
- They are used in culinary dishes, especially during the holiday season.

Pomegranate Seeds (Punica granatum):

- Pomegranate seeds, or arils, are prized for their sweet and juicy texture.
- They are packed with antioxidants, particularly punicalagins, which may have heart-protective effects.
- Pomegranate seeds are used in salads, desserts, and as a garnish for various dishes.
- Pomegranate juice is consumed for its potential cardiovascular and anti-inflammatory benefits.

These seeds and berries offer a wide array of culinary and nutritional advantages. They can be integrated into daily meals, snacks, and beverages to enhance flavor and provide potential health benefits. Whether you're enjoying them for their unique tastes or harnessing their nutritional value, these natural foods have a lot to offer in supporting overall well-being.

Chapter 50: Bark and Resins: From Cinnamon to Myrrh

Bark and resins from trees and plants have been valued for their aromatic and therapeutic properties throughout history. In this chapter, we delve into some noteworthy examples of bark and resins, including Cinnamon, Frankincense, and Myrrh, exploring their diverse uses and potential health benefits.

1. Cinnamon (Cinnamomum verum):

- Cinnamon, derived from the inner bark of Cinnamomum trees, is prized for its sweet and spicy flavor.
- It is used as a culinary spice, adding warmth and depth to both sweet and savory dishes.
- Cinnamon is rich in antioxidants and has anti-inflammatory properties.
- It may help regulate blood sugar levels and improve insulin sensitivity.
- Cinnamon essential oil is used in aromatherapy for its uplifting and invigorating scent.

2. Frankincense (Boswellia sacra):

- Frankincense resin is obtained from the Boswellia tree and has been used for its ceremonial and medicinal significance.
- It is traditionally burned as incense in spiritual and religious rituals.
- Frankincense essential oil is prized for its calming and grounding effects in aromatherapy.
- It may have anti-inflammatory properties and is used topically for various skin conditions.
- Frankincense resin can be consumed in herbal teas for potential health benefits.

3. Myrrh (Commiphora myrrha):

- Myrrh resin, sourced from the Commiphora tree, has a long history of use in traditional medicine.
- It is often used as an incense and as an ingredient in perfumes.
- Myrrh has antimicrobial and anti-inflammatory properties.
- It is used topically for wound healing and to soothe oral and throat irritations.
- Myrrh resin can be infused into oils or used in tinctures and creams.

4. Pine Bark (Pinus spp.):

- Pine bark extract, derived from various pine tree species, is known for its high concentration of antioxidants called proanthocyanidins.

- It may help improve cardiovascular health by supporting blood vessel function and reducing oxidative stress.
- Pine bark extract is used as a dietary supplement and may benefit skin health as well.
- It can be found in capsules, powders, and skincare products.

5. Sandalwood (Santalum album):

- Sandalwood is valued for its fragrant heartwood, which is used to produce essential oil.
- Sandalwood essential oil is used in aromatherapy for its calming and grounding properties.
- It has potential anti-inflammatory and antimicrobial effects.
- Sandalwood paste is used in Ayurvedic skincare to soothe and rejuvenate the skin.
- Sandalwood beads are also used in meditation practices.

6. Dragon's Blood (Daemonorops spp.):

- Dragon's blood resin is obtained from various plant species and is used for its deep red color and potential healing properties.
- It has been used traditionally to stop bleeding and aid in wound healing.
- Dragon's blood resin is used as an incense, in ritual practices, and as a natural dye.
- It may have antioxidant and anti-inflammatory effects.
- In some traditional medicine systems, it is used as a digestive aid.

7. Willow Bark (Salix spp.):

- Willow bark contains salicin, a compound similar to aspirin, making it valuable for pain relief and reducing fever.
- It has been used historically as a natural remedy for headaches and musculoskeletal pain.
- Willow bark can be prepared as a tea or tincture for internal use.
- Its anti-inflammatory properties make it a precursor to modern-day aspirin.

These bark and resin extracts offer a rich tapestry of cultural, culinary, and therapeutic applications. Whether used for their distinct flavors in cooking, as incense in spiritual practices, or for their potential health benefits, these natural substances continue to hold a special place in our lives. However, it's important to use them responsibly and seek guidance from qualified herbalists or healthcare providers when needed, especially for internal use.

11. Advanced Herbal Formulations: Combinations for Enhanced Efficacy

Chapter 51: Synergy in Herbal Combinations

Synergy in herbal combinations refers to the harmonious interaction between different herbs when used together, resulting in enhanced therapeutic effects. This chapter explores the concept of synergy and its significance in herbal medicine.

Understanding Synergy:

In herbal medicine, synergy is the principle that the combined action of two or more herbs can be greater than the sum of their individual effects.

This synergistic effect can manifest in various ways, such as increased potency, improved absorption, or a broader range of therapeutic actions.

Synergy can occur between herbs with similar or complementary properties, allowing them to work together to address a specific health concern more effectively.

Examples of Herbal Synergy:

1. Echinacea and Goldenseal:

- Echinacea is known for its immune-boosting properties, while goldenseal has natural antibacterial and anti-inflammatory effects.
- Combining these herbs in a formula can enhance their effectiveness in supporting the immune system and combating infections.

2. Ginger and Turmeric:

- Ginger has anti-inflammatory and digestive properties, while turmeric is a potent anti-inflammatory and antioxidant.
- Together, they create a powerful combination for addressing conditions related to inflammation and digestion, such as arthritis or digestive discomfort.

3. Hawthorn and Garlic:

- Hawthorn supports cardiovascular health by improving blood circulation and heart function.
- Garlic has cardiovascular benefits, including lowering blood pressure and cholesterol.
- When used together, these herbs can provide comprehensive cardiovascular support.

4. Black Pepper and Turmeric:

- Black pepper contains piperine, a compound that enhances the absorption of curcumin, the active ingredient in turmeric.
- Combining black pepper with turmeric increases the bioavailability of curcumin, making it more effective in managing inflammation and oxidative stress.

Significance of Herbal Synergy:

- Herbal synergy allows for more targeted and comprehensive approaches to health concerns.
- It can reduce the risk of side effects by allowing for lower dosages of individual herbs, making herbal remedies gentler on the body.
- Synergistic herbal combinations are often tailored to specific health conditions, providing a holistic and personalized approach to healing.

Cautions and Considerations:

- While herbal synergy can enhance therapeutic effects, it's essential to use herbal combinations with care and under the guidance of a qualified herbalist or healthcare provider.
- Individual responses to herbal combinations can vary, so it's crucial to monitor for any adverse reactions or interactions with medications.
- Herbal synergy should not be seen as a substitute for professional medical advice, especially in the treatment of serious health conditions.

Chapter 52: Formulas for Digestive Health

Digestive health is essential for overall well-being, as it influences the body's ability to absorb nutrients, eliminate waste, and maintain balance. In this chapter, we explore herbal formulas designed to support and promote digestive health.

Understanding Digestive Health:

Digestive health encompasses the functioning of the entire digestive system, from the mouth and esophagus to the stomach, intestines, and beyond. A healthy digestive system is characterized by efficient digestion and absorption of nutrients, regular bowel movements, and minimal discomfort or bloating.

Common Digestive Issues:

Indigestion: Characterized by discomfort and bloating after eating, indigestion can result from overeating, spicy foods, or poor eating habits.

Acid Reflux: Acid reflux occurs when stomach acid flows back into the esophagus, causing heartburn and irritation.

Constipation: Infrequent or difficult bowel movements can lead to discomfort and a sense of incomplete evacuation.

Diarrhea: Frequent loose or watery stools can result from infections, food intolerances, or gastrointestinal disorders.

Irritable Bowel Syndrome (IBS): IBS is a chronic digestive disorder characterized by abdominal pain, bloating, and changes in bowel habits.

Herbal Formulas for Digestive Health:

Digestive Bitters Formula:

- This formula typically includes bitter herbs like dandelion root, gentian, and artichoke leaf.
- Bitter herbs stimulate digestive juices and promote healthy digestion.
- They can be taken as a tincture or consumed before meals.

Ginger and Peppermint Tea:

- A simple formula, combining ginger and peppermint, can help alleviate indigestion and nausea.
- Both herbs have anti-nausea and digestive properties.

Aloe Vera Gel:

- Aloe vera gel can soothe the digestive tract and alleviate symptoms of acid reflux.
- It is available in various forms, including gels and juices.

Psyllium and Marshmallow Root Blend:

- This formula combines psyllium husk, a natural fiber, with marshmallow root for its soothing properties.
- It helps relieve constipation and promotes regular bowel movements.

Triphala:

- Triphala is an Ayurvedic herbal blend consisting of three fruits: amalaki, bibhitaki, and haritaki.
- It supports healthy digestion, regular bowel movements, and detoxification.

Chamomile and Fennel Infusion:

- Chamomile and fennel seeds brewed into an infusion can ease digestive discomfort, including gas and bloating.
- These herbs have anti-inflammatory and carminative properties.

Peppermint and Ginger Capsules:

- Capsules containing peppermint oil and ginger extract can help manage symptoms of IBS.
- They have antispasmodic and anti-inflammatory effects on the digestive tract.

Cautions and Considerations:

- While these herbal formulas can be beneficial for many individuals, it's essential to consult with a healthcare provider before starting any new herbal regimen, especially if you have underlying medical conditions or are taking medications.
- Dosage and individual responses to herbs may vary, so it's advisable to start with lower doses and gradually increase as needed.

- Dietary and lifestyle factors, such as maintaining a balanced diet, staying hydrated, and managing stress, also play significant roles in digestive health.
- Incorporating herbal formulas for digestive health into your wellness routine can be a gentle and natural way to address common digestive issues. However, always seek professional guidance when necessary, and consider a holistic approach that includes diet and lifestyle modifications for optimal digestive well-being.

Chapter 53: Blends for Mental Clarity and Calm

Mental clarity and calmness are essential for maintaining overall well-being and managing the stresses of daily life. In this chapter, we explore herbal blends designed to enhance mental clarity, reduce stress, and promote a sense of calm.

The Importance of Mental Clarity and Calm:

Mental clarity refers to the ability to think clearly, focus, and make sound decisions.

A sense of calmness helps reduce stress, anxiety, and emotional turmoil.

Achieving mental balance can improve productivity, creativity, and overall quality of life.

Common Mental Challenges:

Stress: The demands of modern life often lead to stress, which can negatively impact mental clarity and emotional well-being.

Anxiety: Excessive worry and anxiety can cloud thinking and disrupt a sense of calm.

Mental Fatigue: Overworking the mind can lead to mental fatigue, making it challenging to concentrate and stay clear-headed.

Herbal Blends for Mental Clarity and Calm:

Lemon Balm and Lavender Tea:

- Lemon balm and lavender are known for their calming properties.
- A tea blend of these herbs can help reduce anxiety and promote relaxation.

Ginkgo Biloba and Gotu Kola Tincture:

- Ginkgo biloba enhances blood flow to the brain, improving cognitive function.
- Gotu kola supports mental clarity and can be blended with ginkgo biloba in tincture form.

Chamomile and Valerian Infusion:

- Chamomile has soothing properties that promote relaxation.
- Valerian is known for its calming effects and can be combined in an herbal infusion to help with

sleep and stress.

Ashwagandha and Rhodiola Capsules:

- Ashwagandha is an adaptogen that helps the body cope with stress and anxiety.
- Rhodiola enhances mental clarity and focus.
- These herbs can be combined in capsule form to support both calmness and cognitive function.

Peppermint and Rosemary Inhalation Blend:

- Inhalation blends can provide a quick mental boost.
- A blend of peppermint and rosemary essential oils can clear the mind and improve focus when inhaled.

Cautions and Considerations:

- It's crucial to use these herbal blends mindfully, as individual responses may vary.
- Dosage and duration should be determined with care, especially if you are pregnant, nursing, or taking medications.
- In addition to herbal blends, lifestyle factors such as a balanced diet, regular exercise, and stress management techniques play a crucial role in maintaining mental clarity and calmness.

Chapter 54: Remedies for Skin and Hair Care

Skin and hair care are important aspects of personal well-being and grooming. In this chapter, we explore various herbal remedies that can be used to maintain healthy and vibrant skin and hair.

The Significance of Skin and Hair Care:

- Healthy skin and hair not only contribute to one's appearance but also reflect overall health and self-esteem.
- Skin is the body's largest organ and serves as a protective barrier against external factors.
- Hair, though primarily a cosmetic feature, can impact self-confidence and self-expression.

Common Skin and Hair Concerns:

Acne: Acne can result from clogged pores and bacterial infections, leading to skin blemishes and inflammation.

Dry Skin: Dry skin lacks moisture, often causing itching, flaking, and discomfort.

Dandruff: Dandruff is characterized by flaky scalp skin and can be due to dryness, oil imbalance, or fungal overgrowth.

Premature Aging: Premature aging is marked by wrinkles, fine lines, and age spots on the skin.

Hair Loss: Hair loss can occur due to various factors, including genetics, hormonal changes, and stress.

Herbal Remedies for Skin and Hair Care:

Aloe Vera Gel for Skin:

- Aloe vera gel has soothing and hydrating properties, making it effective for sunburn relief and general skin hydration.
- It can be applied topically to moisturize and soothe the skin.

Tea Tree Oil for Acne:

1. Tea tree oil has antibacterial properties and is useful in managing acne.
2. Diluted tea tree oil can be applied as a spot treatment for acne-prone areas.

Coconut Oil for Hair:

1. Coconut oil is a natural conditioner for hair.
2. It can be applied as a hair mask to moisturize and strengthen hair.

Oatmeal Bath for Dry Skin:

1. Oatmeal baths are soothing for dry and itchy skin.
2. Finely ground oatmeal can be added to warm bathwater to relieve skin discomfort.

Rosehip Oil for Premature Aging:

1. Rosehip oil is rich in antioxidants and essential fatty acids that promote skin regeneration.
2. It can be applied topically to reduce the appearance of fine lines and age spots.

Neem Oil for Dandruff:

1. Neem oil has antifungal properties and can be used to combat dandruff.
2. It can be mixed with a carrier oil and applied to the scalp before washing hair.

Green Tea Toner for Skin:

1. Green tea is rich in antioxidants and has anti-inflammatory properties.
2. It can be brewed and used as a facial toner to reduce skin redness and inflammation.

Cautions and Considerations:

1. Always perform a patch test when trying new herbal remedies to ensure you do not have an allergic reaction or skin sensitivity.
2. Some herbal remedies may require consistency and time to show noticeable results.
3. If you have specific skin or hair concerns or are allergic to certain herbs, consult with a dermatologist or herbalist for personalized guidance.

Chapter 55: Immune-Boosting Elixirs

Immune-boosting elixirs are herbal concoctions designed to strengthen the immune system and promote overall health. In this chapter, we explore the concept of immune-boosting elixirs and some herbal ingredients commonly used to create these potent brews.

The Role of Immune-Boosting Elixirs:

Immune-boosting elixirs are formulated to support the body's natural defense mechanisms, helping it fight off infections and maintain optimal health.

These elixirs often combine herbs, spices, and other natural ingredients known for their immune-enhancing properties.

Common Ingredients in Immune-Boosting Elixirs:

Echinacea (Echinacea purpurea):

1. Echinacea is well-known for its ability to stimulate the immune system.
2. It may help the body resist infections and reduce the severity and duration of colds and flu.

Astragalus (Astragalus membranaceus):

1. Astragalus is an adaptogen that supports the immune system's overall function.
2. It is believed to enhance the body's resilience to stress and infections.

Ginger (Zingiber officinale):

1. Ginger has anti-inflammatory and antioxidant properties.
2. It may help soothe sore throats, reduce nausea, and provide overall immune support.

Turmeric (Curcuma longa):

1. Curcumin, the active compound in turmeric, has powerful anti-inflammatory and antioxidant effects.
2. Turmeric can support the immune system and reduce inflammation in the body.

Lemon (Citrus limon):

1. Lemons are rich in vitamin C, which is known to boost the immune system.

2. Lemon juice can be added to elixirs for a refreshing and immune-enhancing flavor.

Honey (Raw, Unprocessed):

1. Honey is often used as a base in immune-boosting elixirs.
2. It provides sweetness and may have antimicrobial properties.

Cayenne Pepper (Capsicum annuum):

1. Cayenne pepper contains capsaicin, which can help clear congestion and improve circulation.
2. It adds a spicy kick to elixirs and aids in overall immune support.

Creating an Immune-Boosting Elixir:

1. Immune-boosting elixirs can be crafted using a combination of these ingredients.
2. A simple recipe may involve steeping echinacea, astragalus, ginger, and turmeric in hot water, then adding lemon juice and honey for flavor and immune-enhancing benefits.
3. Some elixirs also incorporate apple cider vinegar for an additional tangy twist.

Cautions and Considerations:

1. It's important to consult with a healthcare provider or herbalist before incorporating immune-boosting elixirs into your routine, especially if you have underlying health conditions or are taking medications.
2. Dosage and individual responses may vary, so it's advisable to start with lower concentrations and gradually increase as needed.

12. Holistic Approaches: Incorporating Herbal Medicine into Daily Life

Chapter 56: Balancing Diet with Herbal Nutrition

Balancing one's diet with herbal nutrition involves the strategic incorporation of herbs and herbal remedies into one's daily meals to enhance overall health and well-being. In this chapter, we delve into the concept of herbal nutrition, its benefits, and how to integrate herbs into your diet.

Understanding Herbal Nutrition:

Herbal nutrition goes beyond traditional dietary choices and includes the mindful inclusion of herbs, spices, and herbal remedies that offer various health benefits. These additions can elevate the nutritional value of your meals while providing unique therapeutic effects.

Benefits of Herbal Nutrition:

- **Enhanced Nutrient Intake:** Herbs are rich in vitamins, minerals, and antioxidants that can complement the nutrients in your regular diet.
- **Support for Specific Health Concerns:** Certain herbs have medicinal properties that can address specific health issues, such as inflammation, digestion, or immune support.
- **Flavor and Variety:** Herbs and spices add depth, flavor, and variety to your meals, making them more enjoyable and satisfying.

Incorporating Herbs into Your Diet:

- **Herbal Teas:** Replace or complement your usual beverages with herbal teas. For example, peppermint tea can aid digestion, while chamomile tea promotes relaxation.
- **Fresh Herbs in Cooking:** Use fresh herbs like basil, cilantro, and parsley in your salads, soups, and main dishes to enhance flavor and nutrition.
- **Spices:** Spice up your meals with herbs and spices such as turmeric, cumin, and cinnamon, which offer both flavor and health benefits.
- **Herbal Infused Oils and Vinegars:** Infuse olive oil with herbs like rosemary or create herbal vinegars for salad dressings and marinades.
- **Herbal Smoothies:** Add fresh or dried herbs like mint, basil, or parsley to your smoothies for an extra nutritional boost.
- **Herbal Supplements:** Consider herbal supplements or tinctures as a convenient way to

incorporate herbs into your daily routine. For instance, you can take ginseng or ashwagandha supplements for adaptogenic support.

Balancing Herbal Nutrition:

- While herbal nutrition can be beneficial, it's essential to maintain a balanced diet that includes a variety of foods from all food groups.
- Pay attention to individual dietary needs and consider consulting with a nutritionist or herbalist for personalized guidance.

Cautions and Considerations:

Some herbs may interact with medications or have contraindications for certain health conditions. It's crucial to research or consult with a healthcare provider or herbalist before incorporating new herbs into your diet, especially in medicinal quantities.

Chapter 57: Herbal Self-Care Routines

Herbal self-care routines involve the intentional use of herbs and herbal remedies to promote physical, mental, and emotional well-being. These routines encompass various practices that allow individuals to take an active role in maintaining their health and nurturing a sense of balance. In this chapter, we explore the concept of herbal self-care routines, their benefits, and practical ways to incorporate them into your life.

Understanding Herbal Self-Care:

Herbal self-care is rooted in the idea that nature provides us with valuable tools for maintaining and restoring health. By incorporating herbs into daily rituals and routines, individuals can harness the healing properties of plants to enhance their overall well-being.

Benefits of Herbal Self-Care Routines:

- **Holistic Wellness:** Herbal self-care promotes a holistic approach to wellness, addressing physical, mental, and emotional aspects of health.
- **Empowerment:** Engaging in self-care routines empowers individuals to take an active role in their health and well-being.
- **Stress Reduction:** Many herbal practices for self-care, such as herbal baths and aromatherapy, help reduce stress and promote relaxation.

Incorporating Herbal Self-Care into Your Life:

Herbal Baths:

- Add herbs like lavender, chamomile, or calendula to your bathwater for a soothing and aromatic bath experience.
- Herbal baths can help relax muscles, ease tension, and provide a calming escape.

Aromatherapy:

- Use essential oils derived from herbs like lavender, eucalyptus, or rosemary in diffusers, massages, or inhalations.
- Aromatherapy can influence mood, reduce stress, and improve mental clarity.

Herbal Teas:

- Sip on herbal teas throughout the day to hydrate and nourish your body.
- Choose teas that align with your needs, whether it's calming chamomile or energizing peppermint.

Herbal Skincare:

- Incorporate herbal ingredients into your skincare routine. For example, use rosewater as a toner or apply aloe vera gel for soothing skin care.

Meditation and Mindfulness:

- Combine meditation or mindfulness practices with herbal elements.
- Meditate in a space scented with calming herbs or incorporate herbal teas into your mindfulness rituals.

Herbal Infused Oils:

- Create herbal-infused oils by steeping herbs like calendula, comfrey, or arnica in carrier oils.
- Use these oils for massages or as natural remedies for skin and muscle issues.

Balancing Herbal Self-Care:

- While herbal self-care routines can be highly beneficial, it's important to find a balance that suits your lifestyle and individual needs.
- Self-care should complement, not replace, professional healthcare when necessary.

Cautions and Considerations:

- Be mindful of any allergies or sensitivities you may have to specific herbs or essential oils.
- Always use herbs and herbal products as directed, and consult with an herbalist or healthcare provider for guidance when necessary.

Chapter 58: Seasonal Herbal Rituals

Seasonal herbal rituals are intentional practices that align with the changing seasons to promote well-being, harmony with nature, and a deeper connection to the natural world. These rituals draw upon the unique qualities of each season and incorporate herbs, plants, and traditions to foster physical, emotional, and spiritual balance. In this chapter, we explore the concept of seasonal herbal rituals, their significance, and how to create meaningful rituals for each season.

Understanding Seasonal Herbal Rituals:

Seasonal herbal rituals are rooted in the recognition that nature undergoes distinct cycles throughout the year, and humans can benefit from aligning their lives with these natural rhythms. These rituals help individuals attune themselves to the energies and qualities of each season, fostering a sense of balance and harmony.

Significance of Seasonal Herbal Rituals:

- **Connection to Nature:** Seasonal rituals deepen one's connection to the natural world, fostering a sense of awe and reverence for the changing landscape.
- **Well-Being:** These rituals promote physical and emotional well-being by addressing the unique needs and challenges of each season.
- **Mindfulness:** Engaging in seasonal rituals encourages mindfulness and presence, grounding individuals in the here and now.

Creating Seasonal Herbal Rituals:

Spring Rituals:

- Spring is a time of renewal and growth. Rituals may involve planting herbs, spring cleaning, and embracing the rejuvenating qualities of herbs like nettle, dandelion, and cleavers.

Summer Rituals:

- Summer celebrates abundance and warmth. Rituals may include outdoor gatherings, sun salutations, and using herbs like lavender, mint, and lemon balm for relaxation and refreshment.

Autumn Rituals:

- Autumn signifies harvest and transition. Rituals may involve gratitude practices, herbal infusions with warming herbs like cinnamon and ginger, and foraging for seasonal herbs and berries.

Winter Rituals:

- Winter invites reflection and rest. Rituals may incorporate meditation, cozy herbal teas with chamomile or elderberry, and creating herbal remedies to support the immune system.

Balancing Seasonal Herbal Rituals:

- The key to balanced seasonal rituals is to adapt them to your unique circumstances and preferences.
- Stay attuned to your own needs and the changing energies of each season to create rituals that resonate with you.

Cautions and Considerations:

- Some herbs may have specific associations with certain seasons, so research and choose herbs that align with the intentions of your rituals.
- Always respect local laws and guidelines when foraging for wild herbs, and be aware of any allergies or sensitivities to specific herbs.

Chapter 59: The Role of Meditation and Mindfulness

Meditation and mindfulness are powerful practices that can enhance physical, mental, and emotional well-being. In this chapter, we explore the significance of meditation and mindfulness, their benefits, and how to incorporate these practices into your daily life.

Understanding Meditation and Mindfulness:

- **Meditation** is a practice that involves focusing the mind on a particular object, thought, or activity to train attention and awareness, ultimately achieving a mentally clear and emotionally calm state.

- **Mindfulness** is a mental practice that cultivates awareness of the present moment, allowing individuals to observe their thoughts, emotions, and bodily sensations without judgment.

Benefits of Meditation and Mindfulness:

- **Stress Reduction:** Both meditation and mindfulness are effective tools for reducing stress and anxiety by promoting relaxation and emotional regulation.

- **Improved Concentration:** These practices enhance concentration and cognitive function by training the mind to focus on the task at hand.

- **Emotional Well-Being:** Meditation and mindfulness can improve emotional resilience and help individuals better manage negative emotions.

- **Physical Health:** These practices have been linked to improved physical health, including lower blood pressure, better sleep, and enhanced immune function.

Incorporating Meditation and Mindfulness into Your Life:

Starting a Meditation Practice:

- Begin with short sessions, gradually increasing the duration as you become more comfortable.
- Choose a quiet, comfortable space and a meditation technique that suits your goals (e.g., mindfulness meditation, loving-kindness meditation, or body scan).

Mindful Activities:

- Practice mindfulness during everyday activities like eating, walking, or washing dishes. Pay full attention to the sensory experiences and sensations of each moment.

Breathing Exercises:

- Focus on your breath as a mindfulness anchor. Practice deep and intentional breathing to stay present and calm.

Guided Meditations:

- Use guided meditation apps or recordings to follow along with experienced meditation instructors.
- These can be especially helpful for beginners.

Mindful Journaling:

- Keep a mindfulness journal to record your thoughts, emotions, and experiences during meditation or mindful moments.

Balancing Meditation and Mindfulness:

- The key to a balanced practice is consistency and adaptability. Find a routine that fits your schedule and needs.
- Be patient with yourself; it's common for the mind to wander during meditation or mindfulness exercises.

Cautions and Considerations:

- Meditation and mindfulness are generally safe for most individuals. However, if you have a history of mental health conditions, consider consulting a mental health professional before starting a practice.

Chapter 60: Community Herbalism and Sharing the Wisdom

Community herbalism is a practice that revolves around the sharing of herbal knowledge, remedies, and resources within a community. It emphasizes the importance of collective well-being, sustainability, and the preservation of traditional herbal wisdom. In this chapter, we delve into the concept of community herbalism, its significance, and how individuals can engage in and contribute to herbal communities.

Understanding Community Herbalism:

- Community herbalism is grounded in the belief that herbal knowledge and healing practices should be accessible to all members of a community, fostering a sense of interconnectedness and support.

Significance of Community Herbalism:

- **Accessibility:** Community herbalism ensures that herbal knowledge and remedies are accessible to individuals who may not have the resources for conventional healthcare.
- **Cultural Preservation:** It helps preserve cultural and traditional herbal knowledge that might otherwise be lost over time.
- **Sustainability:** Community herbalism often promotes sustainable practices, such as wildcrafting herbs and cultivating medicinal plants.

Engaging in Community Herbalism:

Herb Walks and Workshops:

- Participate in herb walks, workshops, and local classes to learn from experienced herbalists and share knowledge with others.

Community Gardens:

- Join or support community gardens that focus on growing medicinal herbs and plants.

Herbal Remedies Exchange:

- Organize or participate in herbal remedy exchanges where community members share homemade herbal remedies.

Herbal First Aid:

- Offer herbal first-aid support at community events, farmers' markets, or during emergencies.

Herbal Apprenticeships:

- Seek out herbal apprenticeships to learn from seasoned herbalists and gain hands-on experience.

Balancing Community Herbalism:

- Community herbalism should be a reciprocal practice, where both giving and receiving knowledge and remedies play a role.
- Herbalists should be respectful of cultural practices and traditions when working with diverse communities.

Cautions and Considerations:

- Respect local laws and regulations when wildcrafting or cultivating herbs.
- Avoid over-harvesting wild plants, as this can harm local ecosystems.

13. Case Studies: Real-world Examples of Herbal Healing

Chapter 61: From Fatigue to Vitality: A Journey with Adaptogens

Adaptogens are a class of herbs that have gained popularity for their ability to help the body adapt to stress and restore balance. In this chapter, we will explore the world of adaptogens, their significance in promoting vitality, and how they can be incorporated into your wellness routine.

Understanding Adaptogens:

- Adaptogens are a group of plants and herbs that have been used in traditional medicine systems, such as Ayurveda and Traditional Chinese Medicine, for centuries.
- They are called "adaptogens" because they help the body adapt to various stressors, including physical, emotional, and environmental.

Benefits of Adaptogens:

- **Stress Resilience:** Adaptogens help the body respond to stress more efficiently by regulating the production of stress hormones like cortisol. This can result in reduced feelings of stress and anxiety.
- **Increased Energy:** Many adaptogens have the potential to boost energy levels and combat fatigue. They do this by supporting the body's energy production at a cellular level.
- **Enhanced Immunity:** Adaptogens can strengthen the immune system, making the body more resistant to infections and illnesses.
- **Improved Mental Clarity:** Some adaptogens are known to enhance cognitive function, including memory and focus.
- **Hormonal Balance:** Adaptogens may help regulate hormone levels, particularly in cases of hormonal imbalances.

Incorporating Adaptogens into Your Routine:

- **Ashwagandha:** Known for its stress-reducing properties, ashwagandha can be consumed as a powder or in capsule form.
- **Rhodiola Rosea:** Often used for increasing stamina and resilience, rhodiola is available as a supplement.
- **Ginseng:** Ginseng is known for its energy-boosting qualities and is available as a tea or in

supplement form.

- **Holy Basil (Tulsi):** As a calming adaptogen, holy basil is commonly brewed as a tea.
- **Maca Root:** Maca is often consumed as a powder and is known for its hormone-balancing effects.
- **Reishi Mushroom:** Available as a supplement or in powdered form, reishi is celebrated for its immune-boosting properties.

Balancing Adaptogen Use:

- While adaptogens offer numerous benefits, it's important to find the right balance for your individual needs.
- Consulting with a healthcare professional or herbalist can help you choose the most suitable adaptogens and dosages.

Cautions and Considerations:

- Some adaptogens may interact with medications or have contraindications for certain medical conditions. It's crucial to seek guidance from a healthcare provider if you have concerns.

Chapter 62: Healing Digestive Distress with Herbal Allies

Digestive distress, including issues like indigestion, bloating, and irritable bowel syndrome (IBS), can significantly impact one's quality of life. In this chapter, we'll explore how herbal allies can be used to alleviate digestive discomfort and promote overall gastrointestinal health.

Understanding Digestive Distress:

- Digestive distress encompasses a range of symptoms and conditions that affect the digestive system. These may include:
- Indigestion: Discomfort or pain in the upper abdomen often accompanied by bloating and heartburn.
- Bloating: Abdominal discomfort characterized by a feeling of fullness and tightness.
- IBS (Irritable Bowel Syndrome): A chronic condition characterized by abdominal pain, changes in bowel habits, and bloating.
- Constipation: Difficulty passing stools or infrequent bowel movements.
- Diarrhea: Frequent loose or watery stools.

Herbal Allies for Digestive Health:

Peppermint (Mentha piperita):

- Peppermint is known for its soothing properties and can help relieve symptoms of indigestion and bloating.
- It can be consumed as a tea or used as an essential oil for aromatherapy.

Ginger (Zingiber officinale):

- Ginger is renowned for its anti-nausea and anti-inflammatory effects.
- It can be enjoyed as a tea, added to meals, or taken in supplement form.

Chamomile (Matricaria chamomilla):

- Chamomile has anti-inflammatory and calming properties that can ease indigestion and promote relaxation.
- It's often consumed as a tea.

Fennel (Foeniculum vulgare):

- Fennel can help relieve bloating, gas, and indigestion.
- It can be brewed as a tea or consumed in its whole seed form.

Turmeric (Curcuma longa):

- Turmeric has anti-inflammatory properties that may help with digestive issues.
- It can be added to curries, taken as a supplement, or consumed as turmeric tea.

Slippery Elm (Ulmus rubra):

- Slippery elm is known for its mucilaginous properties, which can soothe the digestive tract and alleviate irritation.
- It's available as a powder, capsule, or lozenge.

Balancing Herbal Digestive Remedies:

- The effectiveness of herbal remedies may vary from person to person. It's essential to find the herbs and preparations that work best for your specific digestive issues.
- Consider consulting a healthcare provider or herbalist for personalized guidance on herbal remedies and dosages.

Cautions and Considerations:

- Some herbs may interact with medications or have contraindications for certain medical conditions. If you are taking medication or have underlying health concerns, consult with a healthcare provider before using herbal remedies.

Chapter 63: Combating Anxiety and Depression Naturally

Anxiety and depression are common mental health challenges that affect millions of people worldwide. While seeking professional help is crucial for severe cases, many individuals explore natural approaches to complement their treatment or manage mild to moderate symptoms. In this chapter, we'll explore how various natural strategies, including herbal remedies, lifestyle changes, and holistic practices, can help combat anxiety and depression.

Understanding Anxiety and Depression:

- **Anxiety** is characterized by excessive worry, fear, or nervousness about future events or situations. Physical symptoms may include restlessness, muscle tension, and rapid heartbeat.
- **Depression** involves persistent feelings of sadness, hopelessness, and a lack of interest or pleasure in activities. Physical symptoms may include changes in appetite, sleep disturbances, and fatigue.

Natural Strategies for Combating Anxiety and Depression:

Herbal Remedies:

- **St. John's Wort (Hypericum perforatum):** St. John's Wort is a popular herbal remedy for mild to moderate depression. It may help improve mood and reduce symptoms.
- **Lavender (Lavandula angustifolia):** Lavender essential oil or teas can have a calming effect, potentially reducing anxiety symptoms.
- **Valerian (Valeriana officinalis):** Valerian root is known for its relaxing properties and can aid in reducing anxiety and improving sleep quality.

Diet and Nutrition:

- A balanced diet rich in whole foods, including fruits, vegetables, whole grains, and lean proteins, can support mental health by providing essential nutrients.
- Omega-3 fatty acids, found in fish like salmon and walnuts, have been linked to reduced symptoms of depression.

Exercise:

- Regular physical activity can boost mood by increasing the release of endorphins, the body's natural mood lifters.

Mindfulness and Meditation:

- Mindfulness practices, such as meditation and deep breathing exercises, can help manage anxiety and depression by promoting relaxation and self-awareness.

Holistic Approaches:

- Acupuncture, yoga, and tai chi are holistic practices that have been shown to reduce symptoms of anxiety and depression.

Sleep Hygiene:

- Prioritizing good sleep hygiene, including maintaining a consistent sleep schedule and creating a calming bedtime routine, can improve both anxiety and depression symptoms.

Social Support:

- Engaging with friends, family, or support groups can provide emotional support and reduce feelings of isolation.

Balancing Natural Approaches:

- It's essential to approach natural remedies as complementary to, rather than a replacement for, professional mental health treatment. Consult with a healthcare provider before starting any new treatment regimen.
- Keep in mind that individual responses to natural remedies can vary, so it may take time to find the most effective approach for your unique needs.

Cautions and Considerations:

- Certain herbal remedies may interact with medications or have contraindications for specific medical conditions. Consult with a healthcare provider before using herbal supplements.

Chapter 64: Herbal Approaches to Hormonal Imbalances

Hormonal imbalances can affect various aspects of physical and emotional well-being, from menstrual irregularities to mood swings. Herbal remedies offer a natural and holistic approach to addressing these imbalances. In this chapter, we will explore how herbs can be used to support hormonal health and balance.

Understanding Hormonal Imbalances:

- Hormonal imbalances occur when there is either an excess or deficiency of certain hormones in the body. These imbalances can lead to a range of symptoms and conditions, including:
- Irregular menstrual cycles
- PMS (Premenstrual Syndrome)
- Menopausal symptoms
- Polycystic Ovary Syndrome (PCOS)
- Thyroid disorders
- Adrenal gland imbalances

Herbs for Hormonal Balance:

- **Vitex (Chaste Tree Berry):** Vitex is often used to regulate menstrual cycles, alleviate PMS symptoms, and support fertility. It works by influencing the pituitary gland's production of hormones.
- **Black Cohosh:** Black cohosh is renowned for its ability to relieve menopausal symptoms such as hot flashes and mood swings. It may also help regulate hormonal fluctuations during menopause.
- **Dong Quai:** This herb is commonly used in traditional Chinese medicine to balance estrogen levels and ease menstrual discomfort.
- **Maca Root:** Maca is known for its adaptogenic properties, which means it can help regulate hormones in response to the body's needs. It's often used to support fertility and energy levels.
- **Ashwagandha:** Ashwagandha is an adaptogenic herb that may help balance stress hormones, which can indirectly affect other hormonal systems in the body.
- **Licorice Root:** Licorice may support adrenal gland function and help balance cortisol levels, which are involved in the body's stress response.

Balancing Herbal Hormone Remedies:

- It's essential to work with a healthcare provider or herbalist to determine the most appropriate herbs and dosages for your specific hormonal imbalances.
- Herbal remedies may take time to show their full effects, so consistency and patience are key.

Cautions and Considerations:

- Certain herbs can interact with medications or have contraindications for specific medical conditions. Consult with a healthcare provider before using herbal remedies, especially if you have underlying health concerns.

Lifestyle Factors:

- In addition to herbal remedies, lifestyle factors such as diet, exercise, stress management, and sleep can significantly impact hormonal balance. These should be considered alongside herbal treatments.

Chapter 65: Recovering from Injury with Herbal Support

Injuries can disrupt our daily lives and physical well-being, but the process of healing can be aided by herbal remedies that offer natural support. In this chapter, we will explore how herbal support can contribute to a smoother and more efficient recovery from injuries.

Understanding the Healing Process:

- Injuries come in various forms, from minor sprains and strains to more severe injuries requiring surgery. Regardless of the type and severity of the injury, the body goes through a series of stages to heal:
- **Inflammatory Phase:** This initial stage involves inflammation, which is the body's natural response to injury. Inflammation helps remove damaged tissue and initiate the healing process.
- **Proliferative Phase:** In this phase, the body rebuilds damaged tissue with new collagen and blood vessels.
- **Remodeling Phase:** Over time, the new tissue matures and strengthens, and scar tissue forms.

Herbal Support for Injury Recovery:

- **Arnica (Arnica montana):** Arnica is well-known for its anti-inflammatory properties and can be used topically as a cream or gel to reduce swelling and bruising.
- **Comfrey (Symphytum officinale):** Comfrey is often used as a topical ointment or poultice to support the healing of bruises, sprains, and fractures.
- **Calendula (Calendula officinalis):** Calendula's anti-inflammatory and antiseptic properties make it useful for wound care and reducing infection risk.
- **Turmeric (Curcuma longa):** Turmeric's active compound, curcumin, has potent anti-inflammatory properties and may help reduce pain and inflammation when taken orally or applied topically.
- **Boswellia (Boswellia serrata):** Boswellia extract can be used to reduce inflammation and alleviate pain related to injuries.
- **Gotu Kola (Centella asiatica):** Gotu kola may support wound healing and collagen production when applied topically.

Balancing Herbal Remedies:

- It's essential to use herbal remedies in conjunction with conventional medical care, especially for more severe injuries.
- Consult with a healthcare provider or herbalist for guidance on the appropriate use and dosages of herbal remedies.

Cautions and Considerations:

- While herbs can support the healing process, they should not replace professional medical treatment for serious injuries or fractures.
- Allergic reactions to herbs can occur, so it's important to test a small amount on a small area of skin before applying them to a larger area.

Lifestyle Factors:

- Adequate nutrition, rest, and physical therapy are crucial components of injury recovery. Herbs can complement these factors but should not replace them.

14. The Future of Herbal Medicine: Emerging Trends and Research

Chapter 66: Advancements in Herbal Research Methodologies

As interest in herbal medicine grows and scientific inquiry into the efficacy and safety of herbal remedies continues, advancements in research methodologies are essential. In this chapter, we'll explore some of the latest developments in the field of herbal research, focusing on how scientists are refining their methods to better understand the potential benefits and risks of herbal treatments.

Evolution of Herbal Research:

Herbal medicine has a long history of use across various cultures, but it's only in recent decades that it has garnered significant attention from the scientific community. To advance our understanding of herbal remedies, researchers have adapted and developed research methodologies to meet modern standards of evidence-based medicine.

Advancements in Herbal Research Methodologies:

Randomized Controlled Trials (RCTs):

- RCTs are considered the gold standard for evaluating the effectiveness of treatments, including herbal remedies. Researchers are conducting more RCTs to assess the efficacy of specific herbs for various health conditions.

Metabolomics and Pharmacokinetics:

- Advances in analytical techniques allow researchers to study how the body metabolizes herbal compounds. This information helps determine the bioavailability and optimal dosing of herbal treatments.

Phytochemistry and Chemical Profiling:

- Cutting-edge analytical tools, such as mass spectrometry and nuclear magnetic resonance (NMR) spectroscopy, enable the identification and quantification of the active compounds in herbs. This helps in standardization and quality control.

Pharmacogenomics:

- Pharmacogenomics examines how an individual's genetic makeup influences their response to herbal treatments. This personalized approach can lead to more effective and safer herbal therapies.

Systematic Reviews and Meta-Analyses:

- Researchers are conducting systematic reviews and meta-analyses of existing studies to provide a comprehensive overview of the evidence supporting or refuting the use of specific herbs for particular health conditions.

Ethnopharmacology and Traditional Knowledge:

- Integrating traditional knowledge with scientific research is essential. Ethnopharmacology studies the traditional use of plants by indigenous communities and incorporates this wisdom into modern herbal medicine research.

Challenges and Considerations:

- Despite these advancements, herbal research faces challenges such as variability in herbal preparations, difficulty in blinding participants in clinical trials, and limited funding for research on natural remedies.
- Interactions between herbs and pharmaceutical drugs are a growing area of concern, and researchers are working to understand these interactions more thoroughly.

Chapter 67: The Globalization of Herbal Traditions

The globalization of herbal traditions is a fascinating phenomenon where traditional herbal knowledge, practices, and remedies from various cultures are being shared and integrated into the broader global healthcare landscape. In this chapter, we will explore how herbal traditions from different parts of the world are transcending geographical boundaries, leading to a richer and more diverse herbal medicine landscape.

The Globalization of Herbal Traditions:

Cross-Cultural Exchange:

As people travel and cultures interact, traditional herbal knowledge is being exchanged. This cross-cultural exchange has led to the incorporation of herbs and remedies from different regions into local practices.

Herbal Migration:

People from diverse cultural backgrounds often bring their herbal traditions with them when they migrate to new countries. This has led to the availability and integration of herbs from around the world in different regions.

Scientific Validation:

As herbal remedies gain recognition and scientific validation, their use spreads beyond their places of origin. For example, herbs like turmeric from India and ginseng from Asia have gained global popularity due to their proven health benefits.

Global Marketplace:

The rise of e-commerce and international trade has made herbs and herbal products from different regions more accessible to consumers worldwide. This has facilitated the globalization of herbal traditions.

Integration with Conventional Medicine:

In some cases, herbal traditions have been integrated into conventional medical systems. For instance, traditional Chinese medicine and Ayurveda are gaining recognition and being used alongside Western medicine.

Challenges and Considerations:

The globalization of herbal traditions also presents challenges, including issues of quality control, safety, and sustainability. Ensuring that herbs are sourced responsibly and that traditional knowledge is respected is crucial.

Cultural appropriation is a concern, and it's essential to approach the integration of herbal traditions with sensitivity and respect for the cultures from which they originate.

Benefits of Globalization of Herbal Traditions:

Diverse Herbal Options:

People now have access to a wider variety of herbs and remedies from different parts of the world, providing more choices for their healthcare needs.

Holistic Healthcare Practices:

The integration of herbal traditions from different cultures contributes to a more holistic approach to healthcare, addressing the physical, emotional, and spiritual aspects of well-being.

Exchange of Knowledge:

The globalization of herbal traditions encourages the exchange of knowledge and fosters a greater understanding of the healing properties of plants and herbs from diverse ecosystems.

Chapter 68: Sustainability and Ethical Harvesting

Sustainability and ethical harvesting are critical considerations in the world of herbal medicine. As the demand for herbal remedies grows, it's essential to ensure that we harvest and utilize plants in a way that preserves both their populations and the ecosystems they inhabit. In this chapter, we will delve into the importance of sustainability and ethical practices in herbal medicine.

The Importance of Sustainability:

Preserving Plant Populations:

Overharvesting of wild plants can lead to population declines or even extinction. Sustainable harvesting practices aim to maintain plant populations for future generations.

Ecosystem Health:

Plants are integral to ecosystems, providing habitat and sustenance for various species. Sustainable harvesting ensures the health of these ecosystems.

Cultural Preservation:

Many indigenous cultures have deep-rooted relationships with specific plants. Sustainable practices respect and support these cultural traditions.

Ethical Harvesting Guidelines:

Wildcrafting Practices:

Wildcrafting involves harvesting plants from their natural habitats. Ethical wildcrafting includes obtaining necessary permits, harvesting only what is needed, and minimizing disturbance to the environment.

Cultivation:

Cultivating herbs in a sustainable manner, whether in gardens or on farms, reduces pressure on wild populations. Organic and permaculture practices are often used.

Responsible Foraging:

Individuals who forage for wild herbs should do so with care and knowledge. They should avoid collecting rare or endangered species and follow local regulations.

Certifications and Labels:

Organic Certification:

Organic certification ensures that herbs are grown without synthetic pesticides or fertilizers and often includes sustainability considerations.

Fair Trade:

Fair trade certifications guarantee that herbs are harvested and traded in an ethical manner, providing fair wages to harvesters and supporting local communities.

Cultivating Awareness:

Education:

Education plays a crucial role in promoting sustainability. Learning about plant species, their habitats, and ethical harvesting practices empowers individuals to make responsible choices.

Consumer Choices:

Consumers can support sustainability by choosing herbal products from reputable sources that prioritize ethical harvesting and transparent supply chains.

Chapter 69: Integrating Herbal Medicine in Modern Healthcare

Integrating herbal medicine into modern healthcare is a complex but promising endeavor. As the demand for complementary and alternative therapies grows, it's important to explore how herbal remedies can coexist with conventional medicine. In this chapter, we will delve into the challenges and opportunities of integrating herbal medicine into modern healthcare systems.

The Need for Integration:

Patient-Centered Care:

Integrating herbal medicine allows for a more patient-centered approach to healthcare. Patients can have a say in their treatment plans and explore complementary options.

Holistic Well-Being:

Herbal medicine addresses the physical, emotional, and spiritual aspects of health. Integrating it into modern healthcare supports a more holistic view of well-being.

Reducing Healthcare Costs:

Herbal remedies can be cost-effective compared to pharmaceutical drugs, potentially reducing healthcare expenses for patients and systems.

Challenges in Integration:

Safety and Regulation:

Ensuring the safety and quality of herbal products is a significant challenge. Regulatory frameworks for herbal medicine vary by country, making standardization difficult.

Lack of Research:

Limited scientific research on herbal remedies can hinder integration efforts. More robust studies are needed to establish efficacy and safety.

Communication Gaps:

Effective communication between healthcare providers and herbalists is essential but often lacking.

Bridging this gap is crucial for patient safety.

Opportunities for Integration:

Collaboration:

Collaborative efforts between conventional healthcare providers and herbalists can lead to more comprehensive patient care. This may involve sharing knowledge and experiences.

Education and Training:

Training healthcare professionals in herbal medicine and educating herbalists about conventional medicine can enhance their ability to work together.

Research Initiatives:

Funding and conducting research on herbal remedies can help establish their efficacy and safety, leading to greater acceptance in modern healthcare.

Patient Empowerment:

Informed Choices:

Patients should be empowered to make informed choices about their healthcare, including the use of herbal remedies. Healthcare providers can play a role in educating patients.

Shared Decision-Making:

Encouraging shared decision-making between patients and healthcare providers allows for a more personalized approach to treatment.

Chapter 70: The Digital Age: Apps, AI, and Herbalism

The digital age has brought transformative changes to various industries, including herbalism. In this chapter, we will explore how technology, particularly mobile applications (apps) and artificial intelligence (AI), is impacting the practice of herbalism and the accessibility of herbal knowledge.

Herbal Apps:

Information Access:

Herbal apps provide users with easy access to a wealth of information about herbs, including their uses, properties, and potential interactions.

Identification and Foraging:

Some apps include features for identifying wild plants and herbs, making it safer for foragers and enthusiasts to find and use plants.

Recipe and Remedies:

Herbal apps often contain recipes and remedies for various health concerns, helping users create their herbal preparations.

Dosage and Safety:

Apps may provide dosage recommendations and safety information, reducing the risk of improper herbal use.

AI in Herbal Medicine:

Personalized Recommendations:

AI can analyze individual health data and recommend herbal remedies tailored to a person's specific needs and health conditions.

Drug-Herb Interactions:

AI can help identify potential interactions between herbal remedies and pharmaceutical drugs, enhancing patient safety.

Research and Discovery:

AI-powered tools can analyze vast amounts of scientific literature to discover new potential uses for herbs and guide research efforts.

Benefits and Considerations:

Accessibility:

Herbal apps and AI-driven platforms make herbal knowledge accessible to a broader audience, including those without access to traditional herbalists.

Education and Empowerment:

These technologies empower individuals to take control of their health and explore herbal remedies with confidence.

Quality Control:

Apps can help users identify reputable herbal product manufacturers, ensuring the quality and safety of the products they purchase.

Potential Biases:

AI algorithms can be influenced by the data they are trained on, potentially leading to biases in recommendations or information provided.

Privacy Concerns:

The collection and use of personal health data by herbal apps and AI platforms raise privacy concerns that need to be addressed.

The Future of Herbalism in the Digital Age:

The integration of technology into herbalism represents an exciting evolution of the field. As more people turn to herbal remedies and seek information online, herbal apps and AI-driven platforms will likely continue to play a significant role in educating and empowering individuals to explore herbal medicine. However, it's essential to strike a balance between the convenience and accessibility offered by technology and the need for accurate, unbiased, and privacy-conscious herbal information and recommendations.

15. Resources and Further Reading: Where to Learn More and Source Quality Herbs

Chapter 71: Top Books and Journals for Herbalists

For herbalists, accessing reputable sources of information is crucial to deepen their knowledge and practice. In this chapter, we will explore some of the top books and journals that are highly regarded in the field of herbalism. These resources provide valuable insights into the world of herbs, their uses, and their applications in healthcare.

Top Books for Herbalists:

"The Complete Medicinal Herbal" by Penelope Ody:

This comprehensive guide offers a detailed overview of medicinal plants, their properties, and how to use them for various health concerns.

"Medical Herbalism: The Science and Practice of Herbal Medicine" by David Hoffmann:

A respected text that delves into the science and practice of herbal medicine, offering insights into diagnosis, treatment, and materia medica.

"The Modern Herbal Dispensatory: A Medicine-Making Guide" by Thomas Easley and Steven Horne:

This book provides practical guidance on making herbal preparations, including tinctures, salves, and teas, along with in-depth profiles of herbs.

"Herbal Medicine: Biomolecular and Clinical Aspects" edited by Iris F. F. Benzie and Sissi Wachtel-Galor:

A scientific exploration of the biochemical and clinical aspects of herbal medicine, offering a bridge between traditional and modern knowledge.

"Botany in a Day: The Patterns Method of Plant Identification" by Thomas J. Elpel:

This resource helps herbalists understand plant families and identify plants in the wild, enhancing their foraging skills.

Top Herbal Journals:

"HerbalGram" by the American Botanical Council:

A peer-reviewed journal that covers botanical medicine, herbal science, and traditional knowledge, providing a blend of research and practical information.

"The Journal of Ethnopharmacology" by Elsevier:

This journal publishes research on the ethnomedical, ethnobotanical, and phytochemical aspects of herbal medicine, making it a valuable resource for herbalists.

"Phytotherapy Research" by Wiley:

A journal that focuses on clinical and pharmacological studies of herbal remedies, providing evidence-based insights into their efficacy and safety.

"Journal of Herbal Medicine" by Elsevier:

This journal covers various aspects of herbal medicine, including pharmacology, clinical studies, and traditional uses, offering a holistic view of the field.

"Planta Medica" by Thieme Medical Publishers:

A journal that publishes research on medicinal plants and natural products, offering a wealth of information on herbal pharmacology and applications.

Considerations When Using Books and Journals:

Credibility and Authorship:

Ensure that the books and journals you consult are authored or published by reputable sources, institutions, or experts in the field.

Current Research:

Stay updated with the latest research findings in herbal medicine, as the field is continually evolving.

Integration with Traditional Knowledge:

Seek resources that honor and integrate traditional knowledge alongside modern scientific insights for a well-rounded perspective.

Chapter 72: Trusted Online Platforms and Communities

The internet has transformed the way herbalists connect, share knowledge, and access information. Online platforms and communities have become invaluable resources for herbalists looking to expand their understanding of herbal medicine. In this chapter, we'll explore some of the trusted online platforms and communities where herbalists can engage and learn.

Reddit's Herbalism Community (r/herbalism):

Reddit hosts a vibrant herbalism community where enthusiasts and experts discuss various aspects of herbal medicine. Users share their experiences, ask questions, and offer insights.

The Herbal Academy Community:

The Herbal Academy, an educational platform, has a thriving online community. It provides forums, courses, and resources for herbalists at all levels of expertise.

United Plant Savers:

United Plant Savers is a nonprofit organization dedicated to preserving native medicinal plants. Their website offers resources, webinars, and a community forum for herbalists interested in plant conservation.

Facebook Groups:

Numerous Facebook groups cater to herbalists. These include general herbalism groups, regional groups for plant identification, and groups focused on specific topics like herbal gardening or wildcrafting.

Instagram and YouTube:

Many herbalists and herbal educators share their knowledge through social media platforms like Instagram and YouTube. They offer tutorials, plant profiles, and insights into their herbal practices.

HerbMentor:

HerbMentor is an online platform that offers courses, articles, and a community forum for herbalists. It's a comprehensive resource for those looking to deepen their herbal knowledge.

The Herb Society of America:

This organization has an online presence where members can access educational resources, forums, and newsletters. It's an excellent resource for both beginners and experienced herbalists.

The American Herbalists Guild (AHG):

AHG's website provides resources, a directory of professional herbalists, and information on herbal conferences and events. It's a valuable resource for those seeking qualified practitioners.

Considerations When Using Online Platforms and Communities:

Vetted Information:

Verify the credibility of information shared in online communities. Peer-reviewed sources and contributions from experienced herbalists are more reliable.

Respect Local Knowledge:

When discussing herbal practices in global communities, respect local knowledge and cultural traditions, and avoid making assumptions.

Privacy and Security:

Be mindful of the information you share online, and consider privacy settings on social media and community forums.

Continual Learning:

Online platforms are excellent for learning, but they should complement, not replace, hands-on learning and mentorship.

Chapter 73: Finding and Vetting Quality Herbal Suppliers

When practicing herbalism, sourcing high-quality herbs and botanicals is essential for safety and effectiveness. In this chapter, we will explore the process of finding and vetting quality herbal suppliers to ensure you have access to herbs that meet your standards.

Finding Herbal Suppliers:

Local Health Food Stores:

Many health food stores carry a selection of dried herbs and herbal products. Visit these stores to explore their offerings.

Online Herbal Stores:

Numerous online herbal stores offer a wide variety of herbs, tinctures, and herbal products. Ensure the store has a good reputation and provides detailed information about their products.

Local Farmers' Markets:

Farmers' markets often feature vendors who sell fresh herbs and herbal products. This is an excellent way to support local growers.

Bulk Herb Suppliers:

Some suppliers specialize in selling bulk herbs to herbalists and herbal businesses. These suppliers may offer a broader selection and competitive prices.

Wildcrafting and Growing Your Herbs:

Consider growing your herbs or responsibly wildcrafting them if you have the knowledge and access to suitable areas.

Vetting Herbal Suppliers:

Reputation and Reviews:

Look for reviews and testimonials from other herbalists or customers who have purchased from the supplier. A positive reputation is a good indicator of quality.

Transparency:

The supplier should provide detailed information about the herbs, including their botanical names, origins, and any testing they undergo.

Quality Control and Testing:

Inquire about the supplier's quality control measures and whether they conduct testing for contaminants, such as heavy metals and pesticides.

Sustainability Practices:

If sustainability is a concern, ask about the supplier's ethical and environmental practices, especially if they source wildcrafted herbs.

Customer Support:

Good customer support and communication are important. The supplier should be responsive to inquiries and address any concerns.

Certifications:

Some suppliers may have certifications, such as organic or fair trade, which can indicate their commitment to quality and ethical sourcing.

Sample Orders:

Before making large purchases, consider placing a small sample order to assess the quality of the herbs and the supplier's service.

Ethical Considerations:

Sustainability:

Choose suppliers who prioritize sustainable and ethical practices in herb harvesting and sourcing.

Cultural Sensitivity:

Be respectful of cultural traditions and avoid purchasing herbs that may be sacred or endangered in certain cultures.

Fair Trade:

Whenever possible, support fair trade practices that ensure equitable compensation to growers and harvesters.

Chapter 74: Herbal Education and Certification Programs

Herbal education and certification programs are essential for individuals who wish to deepen their knowledge and expertise in herbalism. In this chapter, we will explore the various options available for herbal education, including formal programs, workshops, and certifications.

Formal Herbal Education Programs:

Herbalism Degree Programs:

Some universities and colleges offer formal degree programs in herbalism or botanical medicine. These programs provide in-depth training in herbal theory, practice, and plant identification.

Herbal Apprenticeships:

Herbal apprenticeships are immersive, hands-on programs where students work closely with experienced herbalists. These apprenticeships offer a traditional way of learning herbalism and often include fieldwork and plant identification.

Online Herbal Schools:

Many reputable online herbal schools provide comprehensive courses in herbalism. These programs cover topics like materia medica, herbal preparations, and clinical skills.

Herbal Workshops and Seminars:

Short-term workshops and seminars offer focused learning experiences on specific herbal topics. They are a great way to gain knowledge without committing to a long-term program.

Certification and Credentialing:

Certified Herbalist (CH):

The American Herbalists Guild (AHG) offers a Certified Herbalist credential for those who meet specific educational and experiential requirements. AHG also offers the Registered Herbalist (RH) designation for more advanced practitioners.

Wilderness Herbal First Responder (WHFR):

The Wilderness Herbal First Responder certification combines wilderness medicine and herbalism. It's suitable for herbalists interested in herbal first aid.

Holistic Herbalist Certification:

Various schools and organizations offer holistic herbalist certifications, which cover a broad range of herbal knowledge and skills.

Choosing an Herbal Education Program:

Goals and Interests:

Consider your goals. Are you interested in clinical practice, wildcrafting, or simply using herbs for personal health? Choose a program aligned with your interests.

Accreditation:

Ensure that the program or school you choose is accredited or recognized by reputable herbal organizations.

Instructors and Curriculum:

Research the instructors' qualifications and the program's curriculum to ensure they meet your educational needs.

Reviews and Recommendations:

Seek reviews and recommendations from current or former students to gain insights into the quality of the program.

Cost and Accessibility:

Consider the program's cost, location (if applicable), and whether it offers financial aid or scholarships.

Continuous Learning:

Herbal education is an ongoing journey. Even after completing a formal program or certification, herbalists should continue to learn, explore new herbs, and stay updated on the latest research and developments in the field. Attending conferences, joining herbal communities, and engaging in self-study are valuable ways to expand one's knowledge and skills.

Chapter 75: Staying Updated: Conferences, Workshops, and Seminars

Staying updated in the field of herbalism is crucial to ensure that you are practicing with the most current knowledge and techniques. Conferences, workshops, and seminars offer valuable opportunities for herbalists to learn, connect with peers, and deepen their understanding of herbal medicine.

Herbal Conferences:

Herbal conferences are annual or periodic events that bring together herbalists, practitioners, educators, and enthusiasts. These gatherings feature a range of workshops, lectures, and hands-on activities.

Notable herbal conferences include the International Herb Symposium, the American Herbalists Guild Symposium, and regional events like the Pacific Women's Herbal Conference.

Benefits of attending herbal conferences include exposure to diverse perspectives, networking with herbal experts, and access to cutting-edge research and practices.

Herbal Workshops and Intensives:

Workshops and intensives are shorter, focused learning experiences that typically last one to several days. They provide an in-depth exploration of specific herbal topics or skills.

Workshops may cover subjects like herbal first aid, botany, plant identification, or the preparation of herbal remedies.

These events are often hands-on and allow participants to gain practical experience and skills.

Online Seminars and Webinars:

With the rise of online learning, many herbalists and organizations now offer webinars and virtual seminars. These are accessible to a global audience and cover a wide range of topics.

Online seminars provide flexibility, allowing herbalists to learn from the comfort of their homes. They often include live Q&A sessions with instructors.

Local Herb Gatherings:

Local herb gatherings or meet-ups are organized by herbal enthusiasts in various regions. These informal events provide opportunities for herbalists to connect and share knowledge. Herb walks, plant identification outings, and community herb gardens are common activities at these gatherings.

Continuing Education Courses:

Many herbal schools and organizations offer continuing education courses for herbalists. These courses may focus on advanced topics, clinical skills, or specialized areas of herbalism.

Continuing education is essential for herbalists looking to expand their practice and expertise.

Benefits of Staying Updated:

Enhanced Knowledge:

Attending conferences and workshops exposes herbalists to the latest research, techniques, and developments in the field.

Networking:

These events provide opportunities to connect with other herbalists, build a professional network, and exchange ideas.

Inspiration:

Interacting with experienced herbalists and hearing their stories can inspire and motivate herbalists to further their practice.

Skill Development:

Workshops and intensives often include hands-on learning, enabling herbalists to hone their skills.

Community Building:

Herb gatherings and local meet-ups create a sense of community among herbalists, fostering support and collaboration.

Choosing Events:

When selecting events to attend, consider your specific interests and goals within herbalism. Look for events that align with your areas of focus and expertise.

Take into account the location, cost, and availability of events, whether in-person or online.

Discover EXTRA content

Frame the QR Code and discover a video playlist

for learning the art of herbalism: